T0257679

Blood, Sweat & Tears

Becoming a Better Surgeon

Foreword by NY Times bestselling author Marty Makary

Philip F. Stahel

tfm Publishing Limited, Castle Hill Barns, Harley, Nr Shrewsbury, SY5 6LX, UK. Tel: +44 (0)1952 510061; Fax: +44 (0)1952 510192
E-mail: nikki@tfmpublishing.com; Web site: www.tfmpublishing.com

Editing & design: Nikki Bramhill BSc Hons Dip Law
First Edition: © March 2016
Hardback ISBN: 978-1-910079-27-0
Reprinted March 2016

Paperback ISBN: 978-1-910079-52-2
E-book editions: © 2016
ePub ISBN: 978-1-910079-28-7
Mobi ISBN: 978-1-910079-29-4
Web pdf ISBN: 978-1-910079-30-0

Printed by Gutenberg Press Ltd., Gudja Road, Tarxien, PLA 19, Malta
Tel: +356 21897037; Fax: +356 21800069

Contents

page

The author v

About this book vii

Foreword by Marty Makary, MD, MPH xi

Dedication xiii

PART 1 A surgeon's journey to empathetic patient care 1

1 Blood & sweat: hardship of a surgical intern 3
2 Tears: a 20-year process 11
3 Learning empathy from monsters and muppets 17

PART 2 The better surgeon 31

4 We learn how to cut, but not how to listen 33
5 Let's stop making stuff up! 41
6 A crash course on probability 47
7 Minimizing risk 51
8 How to deal with uncertainty 59
9 You can't fix what you don't know! 71
10 Individual accountability 79

PART 3 The safe patient 99

11 **The "eat-what-you-kill" phenomenon: how to avoid avoidable care** 101
12 **Nothing about me, without me!** 117
13 **Patient advocacy: it's a team approach** 127
14 **Questions a patient should ask their surgeon prior to surgery** 143

PART 4 The unsafe system 155

15 **From 'blame & shame' to system failure** 157
16 **Why our current patient safety protocols are unsafe** 163
17 **"See one, do one..." — no time to "teach one"** 181

PART 5 The spiritual surgeon 193

18 **Your time is as valuable as my time** 195
19 **How to avoid burnout** 205
20 **What we permit, we promote** 233

Epilogue by Wade Smith, MD 245

Afterword by Ted J. Clarke, MD 247

Acknowledgments 253

Abbreviations 257

Glossary 259

Image copyright 263

Index 269

The author

Philip F. Stahel, MD, FACS

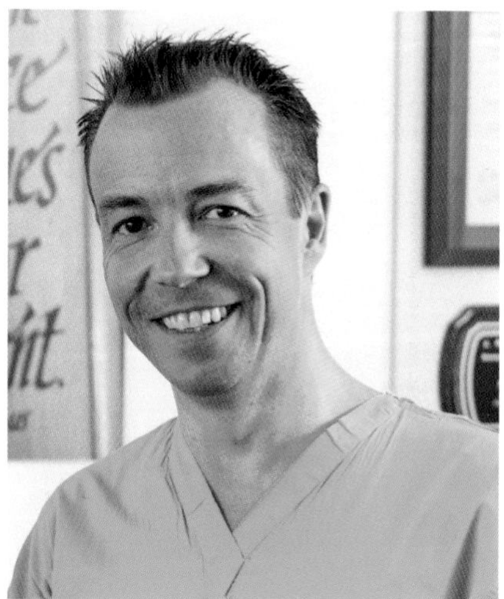

Phil Stahel is a dual US-Swiss citizen who grew up in Milan, Italy, and trained at Medical School of the University of Zurich, Switzerland. Phil completed postgraduate training at the University of Alabama in Birmingham, AL, and at the Charité University Medical Center in Berlin, Germany. He is board certified in general surgery and trauma surgery. For the past 10 years, Phil has been working as an orthopaedic trauma surgeon at Denver Health, the regional safety net hospital and level 1 trauma center in Colorado. He is the founding editor of the peer-reviewed open-access journal *Patient Safety in Surgery* and editor of a medical textbook under the same title. Phil enjoys reading, writing, cooking, and engaging in discussion and debate. He also loves to sail, backpack, ski the Rocky Mountains, and go for runs with his dog Hector. Phil currently lives with his family in Denver, Colorado.

About this book

Blood, Sweat & Tears has been 20 years in the making.

Twenty long years that encompass everything between my first horrific experiences as a rookie surgical intern in 1994 to a recent preventable patient death on the ward of our safety net hospital in 2014.

They say the journey is the destination.

And for me, there have been many stops and starts on my way to writing this particular journey. After fitful attempts at pulling it all together, I finally had my 'moment of truth' while sipping a chilled glass of Greco di Tufo at the Fornillo beach in Positano, the heart of Italy's endlessly inspiring Amalfi coast.

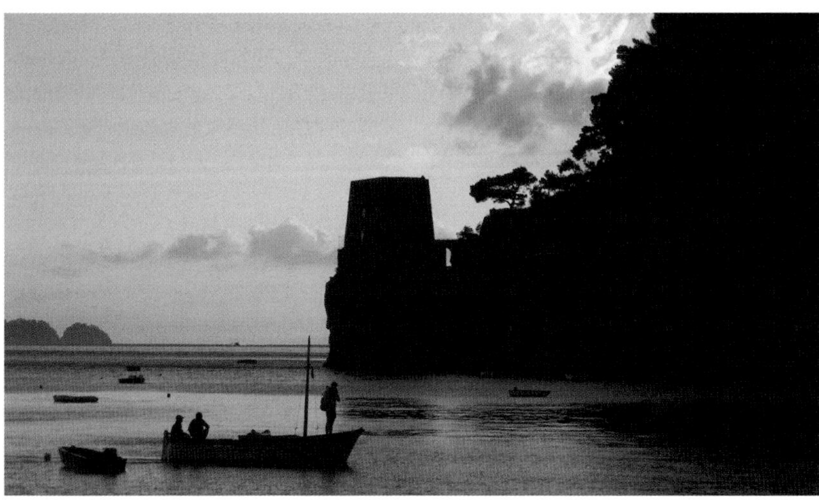

As I listened to the waves crash and watched the fishermen's boats glide into port, it finally dawned on me: I had the ethical and spiritual obligation. The obligation to put pen to paper and summarize my personal experience so that I might possibly shorten the 20-year learning curve for future generations of young surgeons.

Ironically, my endeavor almost fell victim to a 'near-miss' complication. I started looking into publishers in 2014. My first target was TFM, a small medical publisher in the UK. One of their bestselling books, *Top Knife — The Art and Craft of Trauma Surgery*, had been my favorite medical read for many years.

After I returned from Positano, I sent an email to the senior editor at TFM, Nikki Bramhill.

I never heard back.

More than 3 months later, I realized by pure accident that Nikki's timely reply had fallen victim to my pragmatic approach to dealing with the flood of emails in my inbox (see Chapter 19). As I was emptying my 'deleted items' folder in Outlook, I recognized Nikki's lost email just before clicking the delete button.

What are the odds?

How often do any of us look at old emails prior to emptying the 'deleted items' folder?

Close to *never* is my guess.

I immediately drafted an apologetic email to Nikki under the assumption that I had been black-listed as one of those unreliable guys who likely wouldn't adhere to future deadlines. Thanks to Nikki's lenience and apparent empathy for authors, I signed the contract with TFM a few weeks later.

Thanks Nikki for giving me a second chance!

From: Nikki Bramhill [mailto:nikki@tfmpublishing.com]
Sent: Wednesday, September 17, 2014 12:40 PM
To: Stahel, Philip F MD
Subject: Re: RE: Re: Book project proposal

Dear Dr Stahel,

No problem! By all means send me some details of your book proposal. We can then have a chat on the phone.

All best. Nikki

From: Stahel, Philip F MD
Sent: Wednesday, September 17, 2014 5:49 AM
To: Nikki Bramhill [mailto:nikki@tfmpublishing.com]
Subject: RE: Re: Book project proposal

Dear Nikki

I am extremely sorry that I missed your previous e-mail in response to my inquiry earlier this summer… Your message must have vanished in the flood of my daily inbox, and I just saw it as I was cleaning up some previous correspondence… are you still interested in hearing about the project? It's probably best to chat informally on the phone, if that works?Thanks so much, and apologies again for the delay in getting back to you! Cheers, Phil

From: Nikki Bramhill [mailto:nikki@tfmpublishing.com]
Sent: Monday, June 02, 2014 3:45 PM
To: Stahel, Philip F MD
Subject: Re: Book project proposal

Dear Dr Stahel,

Many thanks for your email. Yes please forward me details of your book proposal. I'd be happy to take a look.

All best. Nikki

Nikki Bramhill
Director, TFM publishing

From: Stahel, Philip F MD
To: info@tfmpublishing.com
Sent: Thursday, May 29, 2014 9:44 PM
Subject: Book project proposal

Dear Ladies and Gentlemen
I would like to inquire if there is an opportunity to discuss a new project proposal and to evaluate whether there may be an interest by TFM to be the publisher of my new book?
Thank you very much for your time and consideration!
Sincerely,

Philip F. Stahel, MD, FACS

Editor-in-Chief
Patient Safety in Surgery
www.pssjournal.com

All the stories told in this book have actually happened. I describe them to the best of my recollection. The individual dialogues do not represent word-for-word transcripts; rather, they are my interpretation of the spirit of those conversations. The names of people portrayed in this book are real except when otherwise stated.

I changed selected names whenever the context of the discussion may reflect poorly on these individuals; such instances are indicated by a footnote at the first appearance of the person's fictitious name.

All the numbers, statistics and facts presented in this book are to the best of my knowledge and research correct at the time of going to press. I have to disclose that certain areas that are outside of my personal expertise may lack coherent scientific scrutiny. For example, when discussing *empathy* as a basic tenet of patient-centered care, I purposefully chose not to elaborate on the underlying neurobiological and evolutionary psychological aspects of this moral virtue. I rather attempted to convey the role of empathy from a surgeon's perspective using an intuitive and pragmatic approach.

Citations from the published literature have been limited to a few essential sources that I believed were pertinent to corroborate the content being discussed. The quotes from other sources include a citation and reprint permission was obtained for all images and data reproduced in the book.

Philip F. Stahel, MD, FACS
Director, Department of Orthopedics
Denver Health Medical Center
Denver, Colorado, USA

Professor of Orthopedics and Neurosurgery
University of Colorado (CU)
School of Medicine
Colorado, USA

Editor-in-Chief, *Patient Safety in Surgery*

Foreword

By Marty Makary, MD, MPH [1]

As surgeons, we are taught to master technical skills. And those dominate our training. But non-technical skills (e.g. communicating effectively, coordinating care, and assessing appropriateness) are at the core of sound medicine and not a part of our decade-long boot camp. We train by throwing thousands of stitches with almost no instruction on how to break bad news, individualize care, know our limits, or challenge our traditions. *Blood, Sweat & Tears* colorfully describes why these non-technical (behavioral) skills are as central to achieving a great health care system.

We attract great talent in medicine, but studies show that most physicians will become frustrated and exhibit burnout. I firmly believe that we have good people working in a tough system — a system that today needs a scientific evaluation as rigorous as the one performed on the human genome.

Despite tremendous advances in American medicine, the most dangerous procedure in the ER today is a patient *handoff.* And preventable harm stemming from variations in medical quality remains endemic. Specifically, the magnitude of the problem of unintentionally harming patients in the process of trying to help them is now coming to light with a growing body of research. These new insights are exposing our fragmented system's collateral damage — which is so common that it may be the barrier prohibiting our health care system from advancing to the next level. On a nationwide scale, medical errors of all types

[1] Marty Makary is Professor of Surgery and Health Policy & Management at the Johns Hopkins University School of Medicine, and author of *The New York Times* bestseller, *Unaccountable* (Bloomsbury, 2012).

(diagnostic errors, treatment mistakes, system failures, etc.) continue to burden our health care system. A Johns Hopkins study using a conservative prevalence estimate of 247,912 deaths annually due to error, means that it is the 3rd most common cause of death in the U.S., after heart disease and cancer. Sobering, yet not even recognized in the CDC's rank-order list of causes of death because of a flawed national vital statistics collection process. The problem has been under-measured and under-appreciated. As a result, medical research on the problem has been prioritized far too low. But thanks to a vibrant patient safety and quality movement in America, the effort to address the problem has many highly credible messengers like Phil Stahel.

It's morning in America. Because of the call of passionate and uninhibited health care leaders today, attention is turning to fixing the unintended problems health care has manufactured. Over-treatment and under-treatment are now being addressed as serious issues at medical conferences. Attention is turning from surgical quantity to quality; from the next lifestyle drugs to prescription drug abuse; and from putting defibrillators in every shopping mall in America to educating people about healthy foods. We are at a critical turning point, ushering in a new generation of doctors challenging the *status quo*, asking what's best for the patient.

The privilege to care for a sick or injured patient that comes to you for help is the greatest privilege in the world, and a student going into medicine as a career represents a special calling to serve others. Sticking to our mission to keep the patient first, despite new threats of corporate medicine, will be the hope to address our system's collateral damage. It will also remind us why doctoring is the highest privilege in society. While there are no silver bullets to improve health care's quality problem, there are many common sense solutions that already live in the wisdom of front-line doctors and nurses today. All we need to do is listen to them.

I applaud Phil Stahel for presenting a rich compilation of his honest and remarkable first-hand experiences and the collective work of doctors and health care leaders to reduce the endemic variation in medical quality that contributes to the #3 cause of death in the U.S. today — medical care itself.

Dedication

This book is dedicated to all my trainees
(the better surgeons of tomorrow)
and to my patients and their families
– past, present and future.

PART 1

A surgeon's journey to empathetic patient care

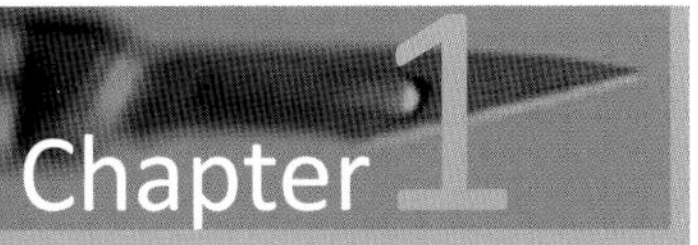

Blood & sweat: hardship of a surgical intern

Part 1

"There are many forces coming together to harm or even kill the patient — their physician should not be one of them."

Arnold S. Relman, MD (1923-2014)
Editor Emeritus
The New England Journal of Medicine

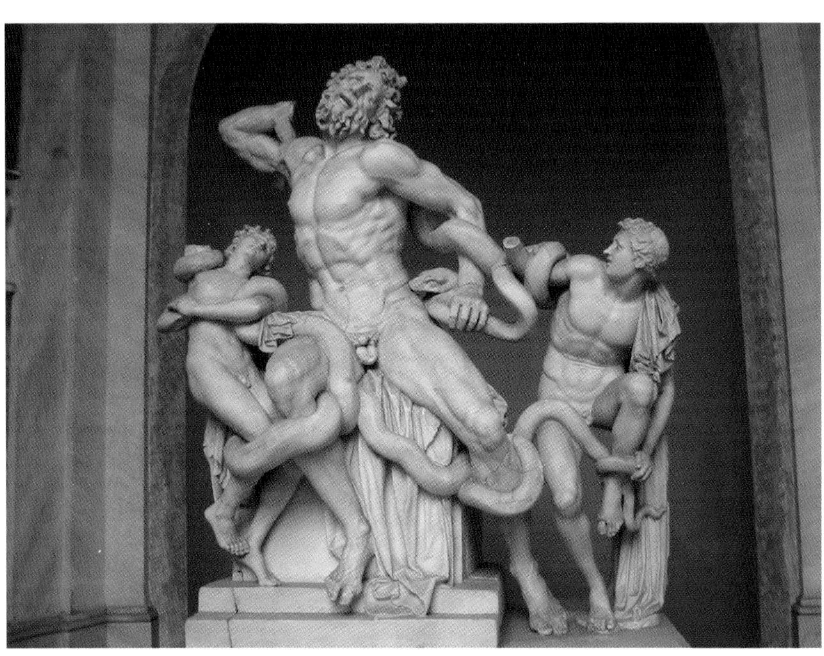

January 10th, 1994

Drip, drip, drip...

Bright red blood fell in large droplets from a red rubber Jackson-Pratt drain into a collection bag hanging beneath my patient's bed in the intensive care unit.

He was bleeding out. Drop by drop.

Drip, drip, drip...

I forgot his name within days of his death. I do not know it now. I never learned what he did or where he was from. All I knew about him was that he was 54 years old, overweight, indulged in fatty foods, rarely exercised, and had a tattoo of an anchor on his left shoulder. He'd had an open aortic repair 6 hours prior to my arrival. I was about to start my second 14-hour night shift as a cardiothoracic surgical intern. According to the notes left for me by my attending, Dr. Gassner,[2] the diseased aortic tissue had been removed and a synthetic polyester graft was placed. The surgery had been a complete success. The cursory sign-out sheet handed to me by the departing dayshift intern stated "n.t.d." (nothing to do) in the column of pending action items.

But now, there was a problem. I could not stop the patient's bleeding.

We had an additional 11 postoperative patients in the ICU. They were all complicated — a devil's brew of heart transplants, aorto-coronary bypasses, and cardiac valve replacements. Most of the other patients were intubated and largely deaf to the bleeding man's painful moans. The 54-year-old grimaced and groaned. He begged, "Please help... please help..." Over and over. Despite the ongoing administration of painkillers it was clear he was in significant pain. The surgical nurses knew something was wrong.

The source of bleeding was evident. I suspected it, and the nurses knew it.

---

[2] Name changed to avoid any resemblance to actual individuals.

He had a leaking anastomosis. All the classic signs were there: abdominal pain from irritation caused by the free blood filling his peritoneum, nausea, rapid heart rate, low blood pressure...

But most obviously, the Chinese water-torture drip of blood.

The charge nurse who only just yesterday had welcomed me with a warm smile and a pat on the shoulder now stomped up with a frown and delivered her non-negotiable request: "You have to call the surgeon." I knew she was right. But, still, I hesitated. Calling Professor Gassner, only hours after the surgery, would be tantamount to my admitting I could not take care of his patient. Worse, it would be akin to accusing him of botching the operation.

Drip, drip, drip...

Three weeks earlier I had stepped aboard a plane and took one last lingering, backwards glance at the verdant mountains surrounding Bogotá. Following my graduation from medical school, I had spent 2 months backpacking through Venezuela and Colombia.

I was hopping from hostel to hostel with my best friend from medical school, Martin. We made our way from Caracas on Venezuela's fertile coast with its colorful fishing boats, up into the highlands peppered with banana plantations to San Cristóbal, a mountain city nestled in the northern Andes. Right on the border with Colombia, San Cristóbal was a dangerous place. In fact, Colombia was a country everyone had warned me about; a country wracked by insurgency, stricken with constant paroxysms of bloody violence. The notorious FARC – *Fuerzas Armadas Revolucionarias de Colombia* – operated on the border and we heard many stories of waylaid travelers. Crossing the border was not easy; we encountered numerous groups of armed men and had to talk our way out of some dangerous situations.

Despite the multiple warnings, I found Colombia to be a country of endless natural beauty. The landscape was picturesque, from the lush Orinoco river basin to the floral explosion of the Amazon jungle. Wherever we traveled, we encountered warm, selfless people who welcomed us, two young strangers, into their homes with open arms.

While in Colombia, Martin and I bunked with a poor family of six in the mountain town of Tunja. We'd stayed up late with our hosts, swapping stories, drinking coffee, and sharing a bowl of *natilla*, a cornstarch-based custard. It poured rain that night. Martin and I slept on the floor and I was awakened by the steady "thud-thud-thud" of water dripping in through the roof and onto my pillow. Despite the hard, cold, and now wet accommodation, I had never been happier.

I recalled that same "thud... thud... thud..." of water 3 weeks later in the cold and antiseptic halls of the largest academic medical center in Europe. The sound was nearly identical but the emotions it provoked in me were torturous.

Drip, drip, drip...

We changed the bag beneath my patient's bed seven times. And still it filled with fresh blood.

Unsure of how to proceed and certain that the man's bleeding was a complication from his surgery, I swallowed my pride and rang Professor Gassner. It was 1:30am and he greeted my call with immense displeasure.

"What is it?"

"Um... I... hello... sorry, Sir..." I stuttered, fumbled, tried to explain what my concerns were. He shot me down immediately, with a crushing fierceness he'd perfected over a lifetime of bending interns and residents to his will.

"Are you suggesting there was a problem with my surgery?" He snarled.

I hedged, backpedaled.

"I suspect it's a leaking anast-..." He cut me off and told me I was mistaken.

He said that it was my job to figure out what was going on and that, most likely, I'd missed something. Surely he considered my appraisal of the situation to be cursory and unpolished.

He hung up before I could even respond.

I didn't know what I had expected to hear. Professor Gassner, like all of the attending surgeons on the staff, was a god. And lowly mortals did not question their gods. His word was *Holy Writ*. His actions inscrutable. If there were problems, I owned them.

I came away from the call even more defeated. The charge nurse could see it.

Drip, drip, drip...

I redoubled my efforts to stop the bleeding but it was useless. I ordered repeat labs, coags, another CBC, and more blood products.

I ran through every scenario I could think of. Every possible test. Nothing was working. Finally, I asked the disgruntled charge nurse what I should do. She threw up her hands, exasperated. "You're the doctor!"

My patient's moans continued. His pleas left me weak. As terrible as it may sound, I was glad when another patient's condition acutely worsened and I had the brief luxury of being distracted attending to her needs. Still, it was only a temporary respite.

Drip, drip, drip...

I steeled myself for the confrontation I knew I had to have.

I paged Professor Gassner again at 4am. Within minutes, he called me back, his voice trembling with frustration. I could barely get the words out of my mouth, explaining the acuity of the situation again. I tried to describe in as much detail as I could what was going on and I asked him politely to come in.

He hung up on me again.

Finally, at 7am, Professor Gassner burst into the ICU. As he pushed past me, I attempted to brief him but he barely listened. When he saw the patient, he became livid. "Why the hell didn't you call me earlier?!"

I would not have a sufficient answer. I was a mortal after all.

There was a joke that made the rounds about how interns took the blame for anything. Attending surgeons would ask junior house staff ironically: "Why did you assassinate JFK?" The interns would reply something like, "I don't know, Sir. I'm really sorry!"

"There is no time," Professor Gassner shouted as he took charge of the situation like a commanding general. "We have to reopen his abdomen now."

I held the retractors while he filleted open my dying patient's gut right there in the ICU. The belly was awash with blood and it spilled in a torrent onto the tile floor at my feet. "Oh my God," one of the nurses whispered, shocked at the sight of the devastation.

Professor Gassner packed the belly with dozens of laps for temporary bleeding control before getting to work on the revision anastomosis. He was ruthless, convinced that only his hands — the same hands that had caused the bleeding — were capable of saving the victim beneath his scalpel.

"Anastomotic leak…" he said bluntly. "You should have known."

As he worked and I assisted, I was sweating through my scrubs. All the stress was taking its toll. One of the nurses watched, horrified, as beads of sweat rolled off my face and dropped into my patient's open abdomen. I was a wreck.

After an hour of surgery, my patient flat-lined. Professor Gassner cracked open the left side of his rib cage, stuck his hand inside and began manually pumping the empty heart. Nothing was going to save my patient now.

The *drip... drip... drip...* slowed, and then stopped.

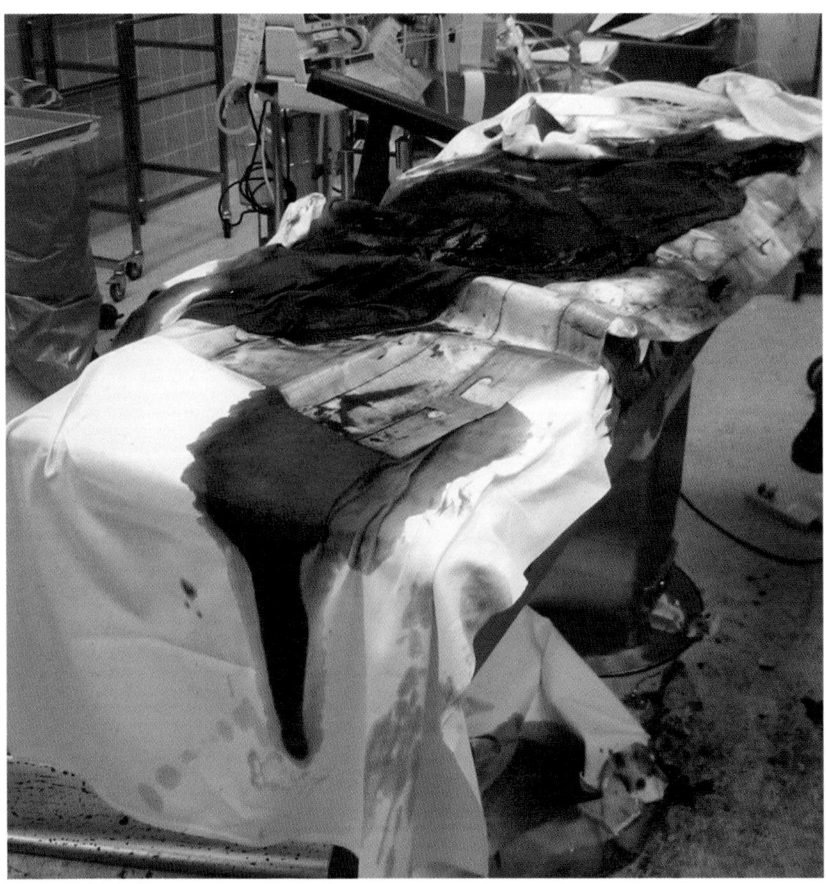

Professor Gassner tossed his gloves and turned to the nurse and me. "Close the belly. Don't bother with how good it looks. Doesn't matter now."

I was beaten, exhausted, and defeated. I sutured my patient up slowly and carefully, with Professor Gassner's words playing on an endless loop at the back of my mind.

My patient's end was horrible. He had been suffering and begging for help that I could not provide. He died on my watch. As I sewed together his flesh, I could not think beyond our shared misfortune. I did not wonder about his family or friends, and the loved ones left behind.

I did not think to burn his name in my memory.

I felt more absorbed about my own miserable situation than about my patient's demise. I was emotionally numb — a robot without a soul. I looked at my own actions from a third person's vantage point. This allowed me to live on and to continue pursuing my surgical training.

I had neither the energy nor the luxury to show empathy.

That haunts me to this day.

My failure still gives me sleepless nights, though the horrific experience clearly pushed me to become a better surgeon, a better physician, and a better person.

It wasn't until nearly 20 years to the day of my first patient's death that another tragic demise made me realize the enormity of the emotional and professional gulf I had crossed since my first days as a doctor.

Her name was Elena Sanchez.[3] She showed me that over 20 years of surgical training and practice I had not only become an empathetic surgeon, but also a spiritual one.

[3] Name changed to avoid any resemblance to actual individuals.

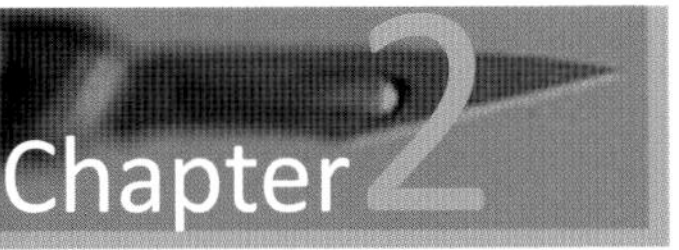

Tears: a 20-year process

"Apprehension, uncertainty, waiting, expectation, fear of surprise, do a patient more harm than any exertion."
Florence Nightingale (1820-1910)

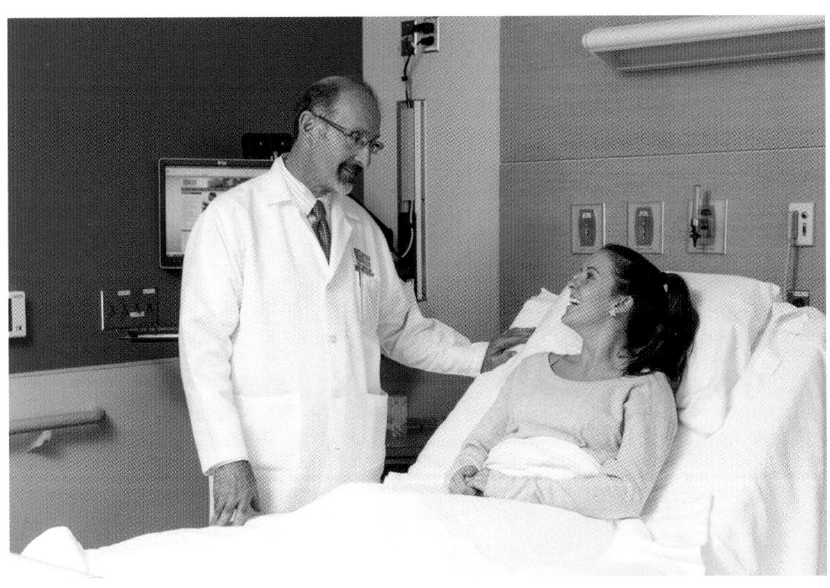

January 13th, 2014

Elena was 35 years old.

Ten years prior, in her mid-twenties, she had been the victim of a brutal car accident that left her paralyzed from the waist down. Despite her terrible injury, Elena had a good quality of life. She was an artist, a painter of landscapes and portraits, and reveled in paint's ability to capture light on canvas. Elena was married and had two young children. She came from a large extended family who stayed very close; father, mother, brothers, sisters, and cousins getting together frequently for BBQs and fishing trips.

Lately, however, she'd been bothered by increasing pain from a bone spur on her hip that had eroded through the skin envelope. This is a frequent complication in paralyzed patients due to pressure on the skin when seated in the same position for a prolonged period of time. Ironically, while paralyzed patients typically can't feel the skin below the spinal cord injury level, they can nevertheless suffer from chronic pain. Elena's increasing amount of pain in a seated position dramatically imposed on her quality of life and prevented her from doing the things she most enjoyed, such as painting and playing with her young children.

The plastic surgeon who saw her recommended a fairly simple procedure to close the hole in her skin and to hopefully stop the radiating pain in her hip. He planned to perform a rotational flap and asked me, as a consulting surgeon, to remove the bone spur during the same operation.

The day of the surgery, I walked to the pre-operative area and introduced myself to Elena and her father. I explained my role as a consultant to her plastic surgeon. I clarified to both of them my minor role in the case and outlined my plan to shave the bone down to allow the wound to be covered by her primary surgeon. I reassured them that this would be a straightforward procedure from my side.

In the pre-operative area, I spent about 30 minutes with Elena and her father to answer all of their questions. I gave both of them my business card with my name and cell phone number, and emphasized that I would be available any time to address further questions or concerns. By the time our discussion came to an end, they both understood that there was little to get anxious about.

Still, Elena appeared nervous.

Confidentially, her father told me, "Elena had a bad feeling about this surgery last night, and she wanted to cancel. I convinced her to get it done, because I want her to resume her quality of life. She's not even able to paint anymore."

I told him that I fully understood Elena's anxiety, and I assured him that our entire team would take excellent care of her.

"She'll be okay, right?"

"Yes," I said. "She'll do well."

Her father kissed her on the cheek, and Elena was wheeled into the OR.

The surgical procedure went perfectly.

As soon as we were finished, I walked back to the family waiting room together with the primary surgeon. We were anxiously greeted by Elena's father and an extended part of her family and circle of friends.

"Everything went well, as planned. There were no intra-operative problems or complications."

I rounded on Elena the same evening and the next morning on the inpatient ward. She was awake and doing well overall, yet still bothered by some postoperative pain.

When I rounded again on the third day, I walked into Elena's room expecting to see her and her caring family. I was astonished to find the room completely empty. My heart sunk when the intern on the floor told me that Elena had been transferred to intensive care overnight. Completely surprised and rightfully outraged, I rushed down to the surgical ICU. I found Elena lying unconscious in her bed, intubated and mechanically ventilated. The nurse at the bedside must have noticed the bewildered look on my face. She turned to me and said:

"Oh, you didn't know? The neurosurgeons have just declared her brain-dead."

My heart skipped a beat.

Turns out that Elena had been given an overdose of intravenous fentanyl for pain control. At 2am the preceding night, she apparently stopped breathing. Global brain ischemia resulted. The chain reaction leading to her death was all too common: a patient in pain, an overworked nurse, a short-staffed ward, a medical error, and a split-second instance of negligent care. The end result was death.

Elena's passing was a sudden shock to all of us.

I was as heartbroken as her family. I silently cried with her father as the team disconnected her breathing tube.

Elena had overcome so much in her life; from the car accident that took her freedom of walking, to the chronic pain that she had been fighting in recent months. To see her die in such a meaningless, random way was all the more crushing. She'd come so far and left behind so much. Two young children to be raised without a mother. And all her unfinished paintings.

Today, I still think of Elena and of her preventable death due to medical error.

Ironically, she had never been my own patient. My role was that of a consulting surgeon. All I did was resect a bone spur for a few minutes in the operating room, as part of a 5-hour procedure done by a different surgeon.

Nevertheless, I knew Elena's family, I knew her hopes and her dreams. Most importantly, I knew how deeply Elena wanted the surgery to improve her condition. She trusted the system to heal her, and the system failed.

I could not help but send my mind spinning back 20 years earlier to my first, nameless patient; the man who died before me, nothing more than an animate piece of meat. He had died under my watch.

Back then, I thought I was an empathetic person in general.

I went to medical school filled with caring devotion and convinced that I would be healing the world. That amount of unlimited passion rapidly eroded within weeks of my return from Colombia, as I stepped into my first responsibility as a healer. Within days, I had turned into nothing but a helpless, overstrained, sleep-deprived intern thrown into the cold walls of a cardiothoracic surgical ICU.

Yet, after 11 years of postgraduate surgical training and another 10 years in practice, countless interactions with patients and their families, and thousands of hours of reading and doing research, it dawned on me. I had finally beaten back the professional detachment, overcome the system-fostered apathy and hypocritical equanimity, to become the surgeon I always wanted to be.

I don't mean to suggest that I finally reached the pinnacle of my career. One of the guiding facets towards becoming a better surgeon is knowing that you don't know everything. As Sir William Osler stated more than a 100 years ago: "It goes without saying that no man can teach successfully who is not at the same time a student." Our eternal desire as academic teachers is to get better every day, for the rest of our lives.

At the core of my conversion to a better surgeon is *empathy*.

I had not been able to save my first patient. But at least I could have memorized his name. I wish I could remember him the way I still see Elena.

In the following chapters, I'll walk you through the steps I took to reach this tipping point. I'll break it down into simple, common sense explanations, objective data from scientific research, and provocative anecdotal examples from the daily life of a surgeon. Everything you'll read in this book is true. I was there. I've lived it. And now I want to share it with you.

So, where do we start? With the foundational concept, of course.

Empathy.

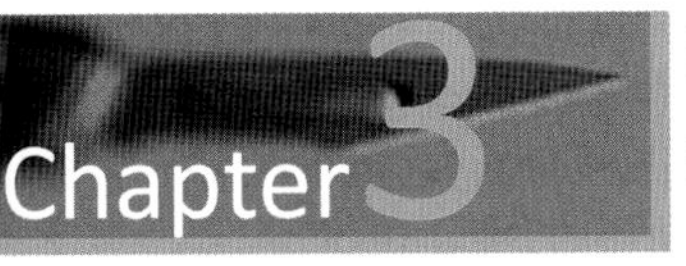

Chapter 3 Learning empathy from monsters and muppets

EMPATHY
noun\em·pa·thy\'em-pa-thē\:

1: the imaginative projection of a subjective state into an object so that the object appears to be infused with it;
2: the action of understanding, being aware of, being sensitive to, and vicariously experiencing the feelings, thoughts, and experience of another of either the past or present without having the feelings, thoughts, and experience fully communicated in an objectively explicit manner;
3: the ability or capacity to understand and share the feelings of another.

We're not as empathetic as we think we are.

We're just not.

We're selfish. We're judgmental. We're stubborn. We're envious. We're greedy. We're vain. And most of us are hardwired for anti-empathetic responses to people who aren't like us. Truth is: most of us are selectively empathetic. I won't argue that this makes you a bad person. It just means you're normal. It means you're human. But I will argue that being selectively empathetic does not make you a better surgeon.

Ouch.

I know. It took me a while to accept it.

We'll get into how to measure if you're empathetic soon enough. We'll also get seriously in-depth on how to become a better surgeon (if you're reading this, you're likely already starting off better than your colleagues). But first we need to define some terminology. When I use the word *empathy,* what exactly do I mean?

Turns out, most of us don't really know.

Empathy is a nuanced idea, a more challenging emotion to get our heads (and hearts) around.

My own working definition is simple and pragmatic: empathy is the ability to understand and share the feelings of another person, independent of whether we agree with that person. In contrast, *sympathy* entails that we completely understand another person's suffering because we have been in a similar situation ourselves. For example, I'm empathetic towards the drug-addicted patient who burned her face after smoking crack with her oxygen mask on, though I can't say that I agree with her actions. I am highly sympathetic, however, to my colleague who was recently slapped with a frivolous malpractice lawsuit. It could have happened to me. That's what I consider the basic difference between empathy and sympathy.

Believe it or not, there's an ongoing debate about whether empathy is felt or thought, i.e. whether empathy is an emotional or a cognitive trait.

In general, we differentiate between two types of empathy. There is affective (emotional) versus detached (cognitive) empathy.

Detached empathy has been taught in medical classes since the time of Sir William Osler (1849-1919), the father of modern medicine. In reference to the Latin term "aequanimitas" (from *aequus*: equal, calm and *animus*: mind, soul), Osler coined equanimity as the idealization of emotional detachment for physicians.[4] On the surface, this concept is very reasonable to protect a physician's credibility and aura. Clearly, nobody wants to see a surgeon freak out under stressful conditions in the operating room or break down in tears after being overwhelmed by a patient's feelings. On the other hand, when equanimity and detachment completely eliminate empathetic and compassionate care, surgeons can be perceived as scripted, cold and distant. They become robotic. Egg heads.

We clearly need something in between. Something reasonable.

"Professional empathy" is a term that I coined over the years in my own practice. This entails providing genuine compassionate care while preserving professionalism, credibility, trust, and respect within the patient-physician partnership.

You're welcome to use it, too.

An empathetic person doesn't just recognize and identify with another's misfortune, but they also understand the gravity of those emotions.

The truth is: empathy makes us social. It forces us to understand the people around us. It is fundamental to how we cooperate, how we grow, how we develop, and how we communicate. A world without empathy is a world of nihilism.

It's not surprising that most people consider empathy a purely human trait.

They're wrong however.

Empathetic behavior has also been well described in non-human primates (monkeys). Furthermore, any dog owner will concur with the notion that "a man's best friend" is highly empathetic to its owner's feelings.

---

[4] Bryan CS. "Aequanimitas" Redux: William Osler on detached concern versus humanistic empathy. *Perspectives in Biology and Medicine* 2006; 49: 384-92.

In a study of child empathy, researchers had a parent pretend to sob, scream, or choke and then recorded their children's reactions. The kids responded as expected, running over to their parents to make sure they were okay. What the parents didn't expect was that the family pet came running over as well. Dogs would put their heads in their owner's laps, eyes turned to their faces in concern. Impressively, recent research even demonstrates a very primal form of empathy, so-called "emotional contagion" in rodents (rats and mice).

Despite hundreds of years of philosophical writing on empathy, actual research into empathetic responses represents a relatively new discipline in neuroscience. We know that empathetic responses are anatomically mapped to specialized neurons (spindle cells) in the anterior cingulate cortex of the human brain. Yet, whether empathy is driven by "nature or nurture" remains an unresolved conundrum. From an evolutionary perspective, it makes sense that a mother's innate empathy would benefit her offspring. For communal creatures in dynamic social structures, maternal nurturing instincts provide safeguards for survival. It's hardwired. And study after study shows that those deprived of maternal attentiveness — think of the tragic cases of children raised in isolation — grow up to have a severely curtailed social competence. It is fitting, therefore, that maternal devotion reflects the first and most primal form of empathy in the mammalian brain.

In humans, the development of empathy is a gradual process. It appears slowly. The primary inklings emerge over the first years of childhood. Toddlers show behavior very close to emotional empathy as their first effort to connect to another's pain or discomfort. When a two-year-old sees his mother in tears, he may offer her whatever he's holding in his hands, like a toy or piece of candy, as a sign of consolation. So where do kids learn it? Turns out, it's role-modeled. If kids grow up in an environment filled with empathetic and compassionate responses, they will automatically mimic the behavior they see. Simple.

And we've known this for a long time.

On the off chance that kids aren't learning empathy at home, we inculcate them via the media. *Sesame Street*, the longest running children's program on television, has devoted several episodes specifically to teach preschool kids about empathy. One episode featured Hollywood actor Mark Ruffalo (he's best known to pop culture fans as Marvel's *Hulk* character, getting green and mean in the blockbuster film, *The Avengers*). He spent several minutes with the red-haired puppet, Murray Monster, trying to explain what empathy is.

Ruffalo summed it up simply: "It's when you are able to understand and care about how someone else is feeling." Murray Monster, perhaps mirroring most children, didn't get it. So Ruffalo ran through a series of specific examples, each one hammering home the basic concept. Two minutes, a few skits, and the message is out there: empathy is good and easy to learn. Even better, kids get it.

So why don't we?

I'd actually argue that we all grow up empathetic (unless we took pleasure in blowing up frogs with firecrackers or were raised in caves by troglodytes). Yet, over time, somehow, somewhere along the line, many of us either lose empathy or let it fade away, unused and unwanted.

Me, I was an empathetic kid.

I'm not bragging. Honestly. Some of my very first memories — around 3 years of age — involve empathetic responses. Most revolved around my best friend at the time, Kurt. Whenever my mother gave me a treat, I would immediately yell "Kurtli au!" (which meant in Swiss-German, "Give Kurt one, too!").

That same empathetic response and same compassionate drive motivated me to apply to medical school at the age of 20. I wanted to change the world. I wanted to heal people. Could there even be a more empathetic ambition than the desire to serve and heal? Sure, you could argue that there are people interested in medicine because they're after the prestige or pay. But there are certainly many quicker, cheaper, and less intensive ways to make money and gain renown.

Regardless, the original empathetic push that led me to seek the rewarding profession of medicine ultimately abandoned me just about when I graduated from medical school.

What the hell happened?

That's what we're going to find out.

I don't think I'm alone in the realization that regaining my empathetic nature was a long, torturous road. With this in mind, I recently ran a formal literature search. The biomedical publication database PubMed retrieved an impressive number of 16,991 records using the keyword "empathy". I was astonished by the sheer quantity of existing publications on what I considered a neglected topic in the field. When I narrowed my search to "empathy and nursing", PubMed retrieved 5,529 records.

That's no shocker, of course. Our society thinks of nurses as highly compassionate and empathetic in the care of their patients. Doctors, not so much. Turns out the return rate on my literature search dropped dramatically, to just 154 publications, when I searched for "empathetic physician".

My heart was actually pounding when I slowly typed "empathetic surgeon".

Guess how many publications came up?

Eleven.

When I pulled those selected papers and read them over, I realized that nine of them had been erroneously linked to my search terms. There were only two articles that truly addressed empathetic care provided by surgeons.

Wow!

So what does that mean?

For me, the take-home message is simple: if only two publications out of 16,991 citations touch on the concept of an "empathetic surgeon", this implies that we're looking for a rare, downright elusive creature. The *Bigfoot*, if you will, of medicine.

So how is it that it takes a 4-year-old 2 minutes to learn about empathy from the *Hulk* on TV, but most surgeons can spend their entire clinical career not thinking about empathy once?

How is it that monkeys, rats, and mice can be empathetic, but surgeons can't?

Honestly: would you rather be treated by the empathetic ape *Caesar* in the popular movie *Planet of the Apes*, or by an autistic surgeon?

Can we really call ourselves surgical 'healers' if we've lost the ability to care?

These aren't new questions, and I'm not the first person to ask them.

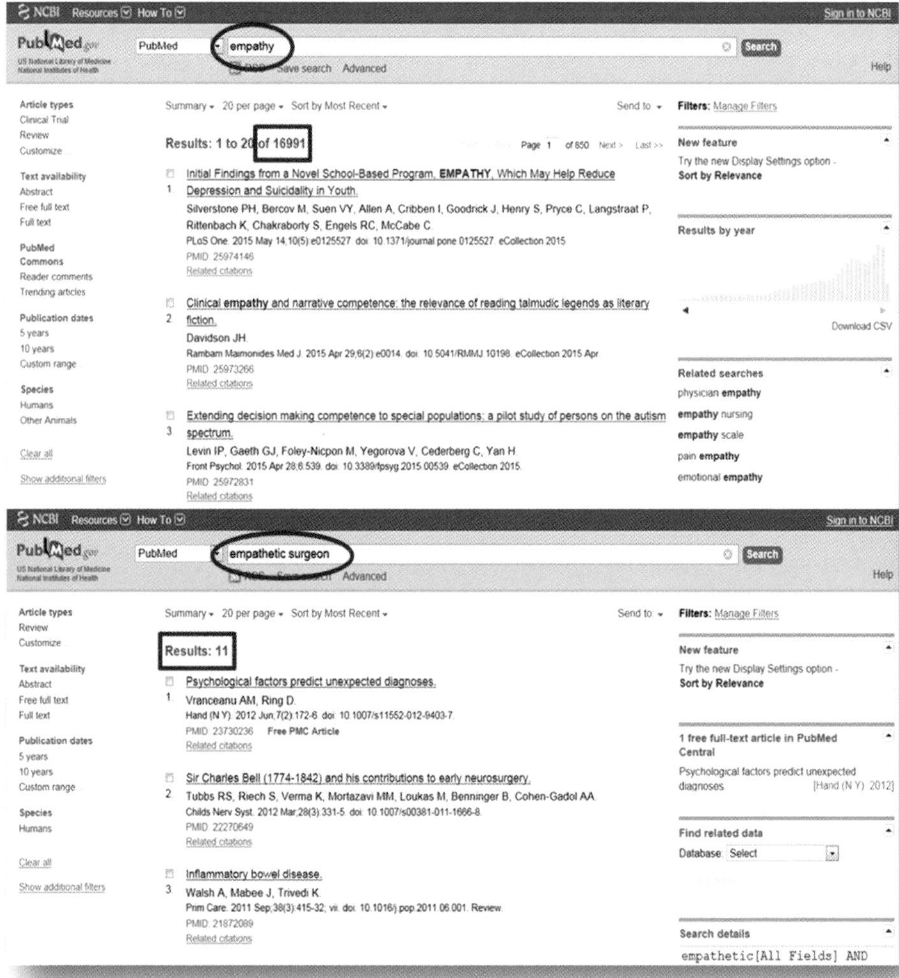

My experience is typical, really. I applied to medical school because I was an empathetic, energetic, and idealistic young adult. The same is likely true for most of the medical student candidates I've had the opportunity of interviewing over the years. And numerous studies confirm that empathy and compassion are the prime motivators for medical school applicants. Yet, longitudinal follow-up studies reveal a sobering reality: the students' empathy rates decline rapidly in the third year of medical school.

There's even a little catchphrase for it: "The devil is in the third year." [5]

This apparent paradox arrives at a crucial time in a medical student's academic course. Ironically, this happens just as their training curriculum shifts from cadaver dissection to direct patient care and clinical work.

This phenomenon is partially explained by the increased competitiveness and peer pressure students experience in medical school; the very same pressure that leads many students to value academic accomplishments more than the humanistic aspects of medicine. In an attempt to hide their own limitations, anxieties, stressors, and worries, most students adopt a stone-cold approach in order not to be perceived as weak or unworthy by their peers. No patient should ever have to choose between a technically brilliant surgeon or an empathetic surgeon. We surgeons need to be more like the *Hulk*, frankly.

Just like kids watching Mark Ruffalo on *Sesame Street*, today's medical students will eventually learn to become empathetic through their teachers. It is our duty as leaders and credible role models to convey the importance of engaged compassion to our trainees and students as part of the routine clinical care of our surgical patients.

So how do we role model empathy if we don't practice it ourselves?

Empathy can't be play-acted. It can't come across as forced. From a patient's perspective, the only practically relevant definition of empathy is a simple "yes/no" perception of whether their physician appears empathetic or not.

---

[5] Hojat M, *et al.* The devil is in the third year: a longitudinal study of erosion of empathy in medical school. *Academic Medicine* 2009; 84: 1182-91.

Yes, my physician is empathetic.

No, he or she is not.

Guess which one patients prefer?

And in case you hadn't thought about it: the patient's perspective is the only perspective that counts. Hands down. In an address to the graduating class of Rush Medical College in 1910, the great Dr. William Mayo (1861-1939) said: "The patient's best interest is the only interest to be considered."

He was right then and even more right now in our current age of patient-centered care and patient experience-driven benchmarks. The fact is, when you're an empathetic surgeon, patients notice and respond.

A landmark 1999 study conducted among female breast cancer survivors showed that just 40 seconds of a physician's compassion were able to significantly reduce patient anxiety.[6] Furthermore, patient outcomes have been positively correlated with the impression of mutually felt compassion and empathy in the patient-physician partnership.

A recent systematic review and meta-analysis of randomized controlled trials on this topic revealed that the quality of the patient-physician relationship had a significant impact on positive patient outcomes.[7] If a patient considers you empathetic, they do better. The bottom line is that patients deserve to be treated with empathy and compassion, rather than to be managed as a 'biological specimen' by their physician whom they entrust with their health and lives.

We're surgeons, not car mechanics.

---

[6] Fogarty LA, *et al.* Can 40 seconds of compassion reduce patient anxiety? *Journal of Clinical Oncology* 1999; 17: 371-9.

[7] Kelley JM, *et al.* The influence of the patient-clinician relationship on healthcare outcomes: a systematic review and meta-analysis of randomized controlled trials. *PLoS One* 2014; 9: e94207.

And you know what? We benefit as much as our patients do: when empathy is considered an essential element of quality care, studies show a direct correlation with improved patient satisfaction, patient adherence to treatment modalities, and a decreased risk of medicolegal litigation.

Physician empathy has actually been shown to represent one of the strongest predictors of good outcomes for trauma surgery patients at 12 months after hospital discharge.[8] New national benchmarks and patient experience-linked reimbursement rates under Medicare/Medicaid regulations may drive a new wave of engaged compassion among physicians. For example, per national benchmarks using the Hospital Consumer Assessment of Healthcare Providers and Systems (HCAHPS) survey, empathetic surgeons will score better on the selected questions related to physician encounters than their emotionally 'detached' peers:

- "During this hospital stay, how often did doctors treat you with courtesy and respect?"
- "During this hospital stay, how often did doctors listen carefully to you?"

It's a no-brainer!

Hold on, it gets even better. Study after study has shown that empathy is directly correlated with a measurable level of clinical competence. In essence, the more empathetic you are, the better a surgeon you are.

While we generally think of ourselves as excellent listeners, outstanding communicators, and highly compassionate surgeons, the truth is we're not nearly as great in these areas as we think we are. As much as we may dislike the HCAHPS benchmarks, we should probably admit that our own percentile ranking on these scores represents a reasonable surrogate marker for the quality of our humanitarian (rather than technical or clinical) aspects of patient care.

[8] Steinhausen S, *et al.* Short- and long-term subjective medical treatment outcome of trauma surgery patients: the importance of physician empathy. *Patient Preference and Adherence* 2014; 8: 1239-53.

But being empathetic isn't easy.

If it were, there wouldn't be a need for yet another book, right?

The fact is, there are many barriers to implementing empathy in surgery and medical education. These days, surgeons are under an increasing amount of pressure. We're asked to perform at the highest levels across multiple arenas. We're expected to deliver absolute diagnostic accuracy and infallible surgical quality under the conflicting paradigm of patient safety and maximal cost efficiency. Not only that, surgeons are also expected to have the highest standards of ethical values and professionalism, required to act as respected role models and dedicated academic teachers and researchers, as well as successful administrators and financial entrepreneurs in an increasingly competitive health care market.

The widespread implementation of work-hour restrictions for residents and shortened teaching curricula for select medical schools offering "fast-track MDs" clearly robs the system of an opportunity to teach the humanitarian aspects of medical care.

I have a friend who graduated from a fast-track medical school program a few years ago. He dived right into private practice and felt disconnected from his patients. Though he considered himself an effective physician — treating their ills, improving their health — he felt there was a piece missing. He wasn't as good as he'd hoped to be.

So he quit. He took a year off, spent his time playing card games (and winning quite a few regional championships), reading, and catching up on the college experience he missed. That year rounded him out. It gave him back his drive and bridged the spiritual disconnect. Seeing patients again, he was a different person.

He listened. He felt empathy. And he was a better physician.

When it comes down to it, we can use all imposed barriers as cheap excuses, or we can use them as an opportunity for change.

Florence Nightingale, the founder of modern nursing, stated that the secret of her success was that she "never gave or took any excuse". The same fundamental pledge should apply to the noble profession of surgeons.

No excuses.

Here's the thing: you've read what I've had to say. You've looked over the facts and figures, maybe even looked up the selected journal articles that I cited. You've read them and you think you're ready to put this into practice.

You're telling yourself: I can be empathetic. I can be a better surgeon now.

You're still wrong.

How come?

Because dramatic changes are never easy.

I often think of Al Pacino's famous speech in the award-winning 1992 film, *Scent of a Woman*. Simple, breathtaking, his character said:

> "Now, I have come to the crossroads of my life. I always knew what the right path was. Without exception, I knew. But I never took it. You know why? It was too damn hard!"

I couldn't agree more.

The path to becoming a better surgeon is just as hard as anything.

Let me show you where it starts.

PART 2
The better surgeon

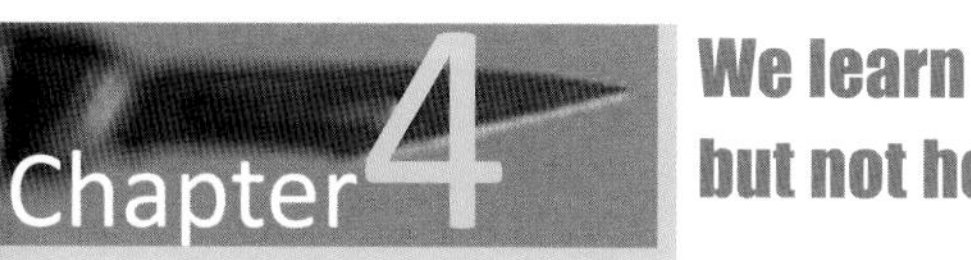

We learn how to cut, but not how to listen

"Listen to the patient — he is telling you the diagnosis."
Sir William Osler (1849-1919)

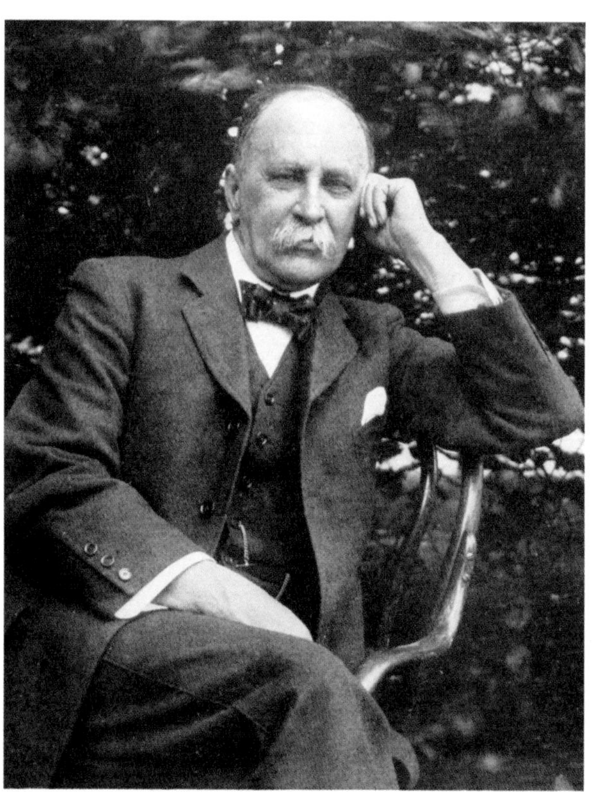

So you think it's easy to learn and show empathy, huh? If a muppet can do it, you can do it, right? Well then, let me challenge you with a truly difficult task: to learn how to listen to your patients!

Guess what?

We don't take time to listen to our patients as often or as long as we should.

No surprise, right?

On average, most physicians let patients speak for only 12 seconds before they interrupt for the first time.

Yeah, *twelve seconds*.

See what that means: if I were a new patient in your office, you'd have already interrupted me by now!

And guess what? The "12 seconds study" was based on family physicians.[9] Isn't it a basic job description for family physicians to listen to their patients (as much as we surgeons should know how 'to cut')? In essence, family physicians should be expert listeners. That's what they do for a living. Yet, the *Family Medicine* paper [9] showed that during an average encounter of 11 minutes, patients were allowed to speak for less than 4 minutes in total. Now use your imagination to extrapolate these insights to a surgeon's office. When was the last time you ever spent 11 minutes face-to-face with one of your patients? And how many minutes (or seconds?) did you let the patient speak without interruption?

Given all this, it's incredibly ironic that most physicians consider themselves good communicators. I include myself. In reality, less than 20% of all physicians have ever been trained to effectively talk with — and listen to — their patients.

Less than 20%!

---

[9] Rhoades DR, *et al.* Speaking and interruptions during primary care office visits. *Family Medicine* 2001; 33: 528-32.

Would you want to be operated on by a 0.2 FTE part-time surgeon?

Or seek counsel for medical care by an untrained part-time listener?

That's only scratching the surface.

Today's surgeons are as technically advanced as they've ever been. We refine and perfect our surgical skills on a near daily basis. And yet we continue to create complications. What most of us don't realize is that the chief cause of preventable patient harm is simple communication failure.[10, 11] As surgeons, we tend to assume that our complications are generally related to gaffes in technical skill or to the inherent risk of an untrained surgical blade 'gone wrong'. However, the vast body of current data support the very opposite idea: adverse events resulting from surgical interventions are more frequently related to errors occurring *before* and *after* a surgical procedure than technical mistakes during surgery.[12]

These errors include a breakdown in communication within the surgical team, delays in diagnosis or a failure to diagnose, and delays in treatment or a failure to treat.

If we truly intend to protect our patients from surgical complications, preventable harm, and potentially death, our success is contingent on becoming better listeners.

It's not optional.

Like you, I studied everything in *pre-med* from chemistry and physics to histology and physiology. In my clinical studies I learned all about the pathology and pathophysiology of our complex organ systems and the principles of how to diagnose and cure hundreds, or even thousands, of diseases. My surgical mentors taught me how to hold a knife and how to

---

10 Greenberg CC, *et al.* Patterns of communication breakdown resulting in injury to surgical patients. *Journal of the American College of Surgeons* 2007; 204: 533-40.

11 Griffen FD, *et al.* The American College of Surgeons' closed claims study: new insights for improving care. *Journal of the American College of Surgeons* 2007; 204: 561-9.

12 Youngson GG, Flin R. Patient safety in surgery: non-technical aspects of safe surgical performance. *Patient Safety in Surgery* 2010; 4: 4.

cut. I learned to safely remove diseased organs, like thyroid glands, gallbladders, inflamed appendices, and parts of the stomach and intestines. I learned to read and interpret an MRI of the brain and to safely maneuver large-caliber screws around a broken spine. I learned to save limbs and lives, and to open and 'pack' body cavities for the control of acute exsanguinating hemorrhage. And yet, in three decades of learning and teaching, and after attending all those endless lectures, classes, and courses, I was never once taught how to *listen* to my patients!

Everything I have learned about it, I did on my own. This is quite mind boggling, as the technique of listening is so darn simple.

There are two essential parts to it: 1) shut up, and 2) listen.

Sir Winston Churchill once said: "Courage is what it takes to stand up and speak; courage is also what it takes to sit down and listen."

Let's face it: the recent global introduction of Electronic Health Records (EHR) hasn't exactly helped either. The modernization of the patient-physician encounter has, in fact, dramatically increased the likelihood of a physician interrupting their patient. Clinicians turn away from their patients to type, interrupt to check boxes, and focus on other EHR-driven distractions. For the most part, the new tools and gadgets have created more opportunities for communication breakdown than they have streamlined and optimized the quality of patient encounters.

Unequivocally, the core principle for building and sustaining a strong relationship with our patients is communication. Open, engaging, and effective dialogue with our patients (and their family members) is paramount to our success as surgeons. You would think it goes without saying that we can only understand our patients if we actually listen to them. There is a famous quote from the world of leadership: "Never miss an opportunity to say nothing!"

I don't think it comes as a surprise to say that, as surgeons, we're often categorized as A-type personalities. We have achieved our main goals in life by being overly competitive; from getting into med school, to residency, fellowships, and academic positions. And just as few meaningful achievements come easily, there are often times hundreds of competitors watching, waiting to see us hesitate and fail, ready to take our spot. So it makes sense that we're not exactly primed to sit down, relax, and spend minutes (*quelle horreur!*) quietly and attentively listening to our patients.

So why would working to improve communication and listening skills be important for surgeons?

Well, let me ask you: How much do you value your career? Your professional standing?

Multiple studies have shown that effective communication with patients is directly associated with:

- fewer medicolegal claims and lawsuits;
- improved clinical outcomes;
- better patient compliance with recommended treatment regimens;
- fewer unplanned readmissions; and
- better quality of care, as perceived by patients.

Who wouldn't want that?

Since this is supposed to be a "how to..." manual for better surgeons, I know you're itching for me to tell you the secret of success; a foolproof way to become a better listener.

As I will elaborate in Part 5 of this book, it comes down to *discipline* and *rituals*. You need to think of it as just another competition. Only that this time it's a competition between you and the former you!

Seriously.

Try this: challenge yourself during the next patient encounter.

Tell yourself: "I was a lousy listener yesterday, but I'm a rock-star listener today." When the patient sits down across from you, simply shut your mouth and listen. Here's a simple checklist for this ritual:

- Sit down at the same eye level, face-to-face with your patient.
- Don't check your watch.
- Don't check your phone or the computer screen.
- Don't think about the next patient on your schedule.
- Don't think about tomorrow.
- Just enjoy the moment.
- Actively listen. Live your patient's experiences, feel their emotions, and attempt to fully understand their story.

Trust me when I tell you it's not a waste of your time. It's the fundamental principle of providing effective and safe health care. At the same time, it's an insurance to protect from the dangers of physician burnout. Listening to your patients will definitely make you a better surgeon, if for no other reason than due to your ability to pick the *right* patient for the *right* procedure at the *right* time.

Let me be very clear: it's really not about the quantity of time spent with the patient. Listening with unlimited dedication for just 2 minutes without interruption may simply 'do the job'.

I'm not making that up! Multiple studies have shown that patients do not correlate quality of an encounter with the *amount* of time spent face-to-face, but rather with the *perceived* quality time dedicated by the physician.

Two minutes of full dedication and uninterrupted listening, including *readbacks* (or *teachbacks*) to confirm we understand and correctly reproduce the patient's story, are more effective for both parties than 20 minutes of erratic interruptions, inattentive listening, and phone and watch checking. If we opt out, we become vulnerable to drawing erroneous conclusions that will lead to a wrong diagnosis and subsequently to a wrong (or unneeded) surgical procedure.

Two minutes is nothing. Think of how easily we waste 2 minutes on less important stuff every single day!

I looked up some random stats. In 2015, on average, we spend our precious time every day as follows:

- 25 minutes traveling to work.
- 33 minutes answering emails.
- 39 minutes caring for our pets.
- 40 minutes on Facebook.
- 4.9 hours watching TV (34 hours per week — almost a full-time job).
- 6.8 hours sleeping.

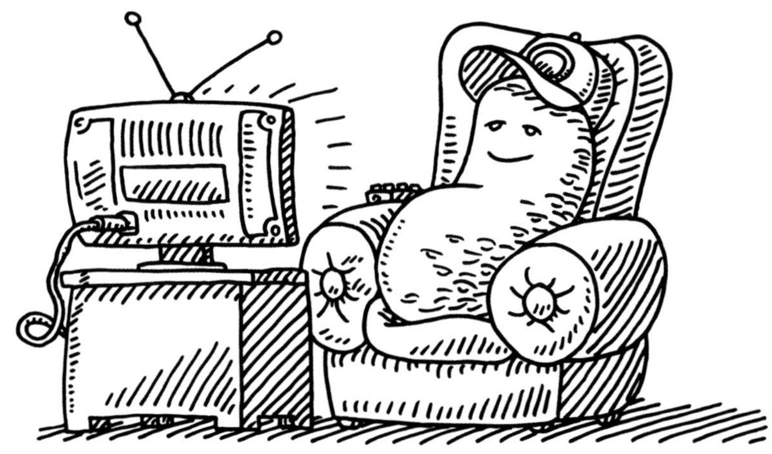

How about a provocative suggestion: let's dedicate 2 minutes per patient to 20 patients per day. We can make up those 40 minutes by signing off from Facebook (an executive decision I made many years ago!), and by dedicating at least as much quality time to our patients as we dedicate to our pets. This pragmatic solution won't even affect our daily 5 hours of watching TV and 7 hours of beauty sleep.

We will become better surgeons by setting our priorities straight.

In essence, just sit down and simply enjoy the moment listening to your patient. Attempt to live their experiences and emotions in your imagination, and try your best to fully understand their story. Of course, this brings us back again to the fundamental principles outlined by Sir William Osler 100 years ago, who taught his students that: "the only valuable textbook in medicine is the patient himself."

All we have to do is to learn from the masters. There is nothing new under the sun.

So you say you want to be a better surgeon?

Well then, shut up and listen!

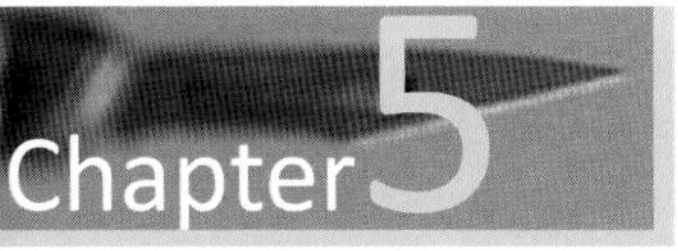

Chapter 5 Let's stop making stuff up!

"When a doctor goes wrong, he is the first of criminals. He has the nerve and he has the knowledge."

Sherlock Holmes, in Sir Arthur Conan Doyle's *The Adventure of the Speckled Band* (1892)

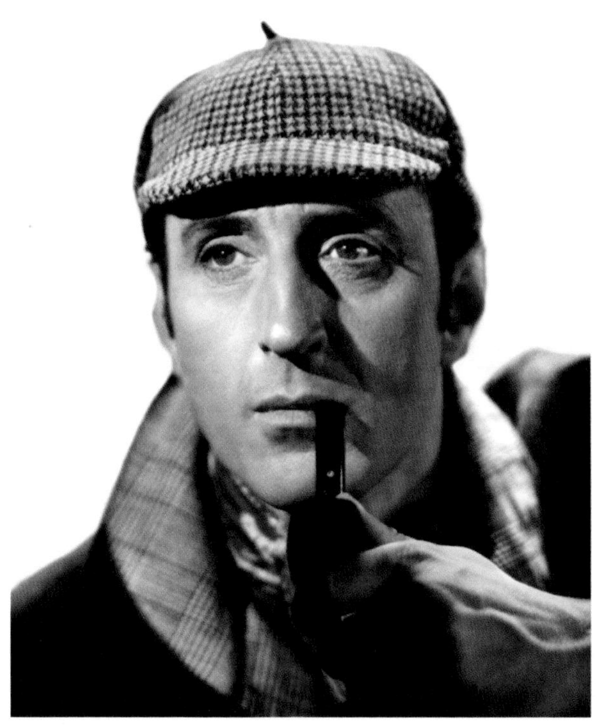

Let me paint a scene for you that plays out in hospitals, clinics, and physicians' offices across the globe thousands of times a day. Mrs. Smith, a lovely 49-year-old lady suffering from chronic lower back pain meets with her surgeon to discuss a spinal fusion. The surgeon is highly skilled, fellowship trained, and has been running a busy spine practice for several years.

Mrs. Smith is very educated and has spent some time reading up on her surgeon and on the recommended procedure on Google and Healthgrades. She comes armed with a printed list of specific questions.

"So, doctor, what's the risk of me sustaining a surgical complication from this spine fusion?"

The surgeon thinks for a second but he already knows the answer: "1% to 2%."

"And what are the odds of a postoperative infection?" She asks.

"As I said, about 1% to 2%."

"And the probability of adverse events or a poor outcome?"

"Again, about 1% to 2%."

"How do you know?"

"I've done tens of thousands of these procedures, that's how I know!"

Sound familiar?

How about we run a little 'Truth Test' and analyze this anecdotal conversation?

First, let's dive into the idea that our fictitious surgeon's complication rate is truly 1% to 2%. How does he know? Does this surgeon prospectively collect and analyze all complications related to this particular surgical procedure (numerator) and calculate the monthly and yearly complication rate in relation to the overall number of surgical cases performed (denominator)? If so, the estimated complication rate of "1% to 2%" should fluctuate over time, and the next patient, Mrs. Jones, should get a different estimate during the pre-operative discussion a couple of months later.

Wanna bet that the answer to Mrs. Jones' questions will also be answered by the magical 1% to 2%?

Shouldn't a patient expect (and rightfully deserve) a more detailed answer, something like this: "My own complication rate for a one-level transforaminal lumbar interbody fusion was 3.4% last month, and 2.8% over the entire year. My current infection rate for this particular procedure is 1.3% in non-diabetic patients, and twice that in patients with poorly controlled diabetes."

You think that's fantasy? Our group at Denver Health collects and reviews all surgical complications, medical errors, and other adverse events once a week in a standardized fashion. For the sake of transparency, we publish a monthly scorecard that is reflective of productivity and quality metrics for all the surgeons in our department. This scorecard allows our entire group of partners to know and to disclose their real numbers and stats.

For example, in 2014, I performed 551 surgical procedures with an overall complication rate of 5.4% (including *near miss* and *no harm* events) and a postoperative surgical site infection rate of 0.73%. These numbers change every month and from year to year. But they are real.

In the absence of an objective scorecard, is it legitimate for the fictitious surgeon in our anecdotal example to simply dismiss the patient with an imaginary complication rate of 1% to 2%? Or else, how does he know? Is he just guessing? Or is it a little white lie to put his patient at ease?

Maybe the correct (and honest) answer should rather be: "I really don't know my complication rate, but thanks for asking."

Would you ever consider boarding a plane if you knew the captain was dishonest about his logged flight time?

I wouldn't.

What if, even worse, the captain didn't even know what his logged flight time was?

That's scary.

Now imagine how our imaginary patient at the outset of this chapter would feel if she knew her surgeon was just making up numbers.

Let's be honest: how many times have you told your patients that their expected complication rate is "around 1% to 2%"? Next time you use this estimate, reflect about it for a second. If those numbers are real, which of the two is it? In essence, 2% represents 100% more than 1%. Thus, the patient's complication risk could be doubled in the same estimate.

Imagine the analogous conversation in a car dealership:

"Hey, how much for this used Jeep?"

"Oh, that's somewhere between $5,000 and $10,000."

C'mon doc!

I can't imagine a surgeon purposefully providing inaccurate data to their patients in an attempt to 'sell' a specific surgical procedure the way a used car dealer attempts to pass off a lemon to a buyer. So why aren't we able to provide accurate data and honest responses to our patients? Is it because we just don't know any better? Well then, maybe it's time for a change in mindset.

Tall order, I know. But stick with me on this. We haven't even finalized the 'Truth Test' from the introductory conversation at the beginning of this chapter.

We clearly run into trouble when looking at the idea that this surgeon, or any surgeon practicing today, could have performed "tens of thousands" of identical surgical procedures.

Let's assume at the outset that an above-average, extremely busy surgeon might perform as many as 1,000 surgical procedures per year. It would take him 10 years to reach the threshold of 10,000 cases. And consider that this is still a mix of many different surgical procedures. Even at an uninterrupted pace without a single day off work it would take a surgeon several decades in practice, if not an entire career, to perform 10,000 identical procedures. Considering our fictitious surgeon even went as far as to pluralize it ("tens of thousands"), we can safely assume no surgeon could ever live long enough to achieve this ridiculous imaginary quota.

The 'Truth Test' failed again.

The fact is: the more we get away with dishonesty, the more we believe our own made-up data as being reflective of reality. Even in my own practice, there's an inherent appeal in hyperbolizing my stats for surgical procedures. I have many times assumed that I'd "fixed thousands of pelvic fractures" and "rodded tens of thousands of broken femurs", with an average complication rate of 1% to 2%.

But it just didn't happen.

The first step in becoming a better surgeon is to know and understand the detailed underlying data related to our surgical performance. And yes, this includes all the 'bad stuff': preventable and non-preventable complications, errors in judgment, technique, and patient selection, wrong timing of surgery, unplanned patient readmissions, poor outcomes, and patient deaths.

From this follows the only logical second step: we will no longer be obliged to make stuff up.

By being honest with our patients we achieve the next level of empathy.

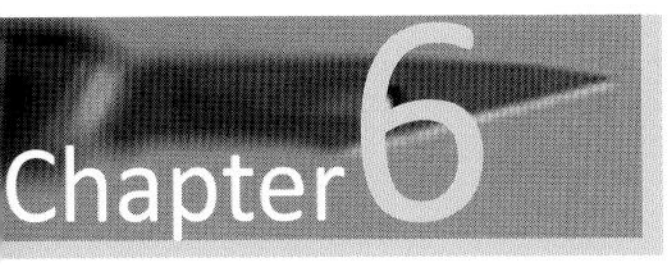

A crash course on probability

"If you cannot explain it simply, you do not understand it well enough."

Albert Einstein (1879-1955)

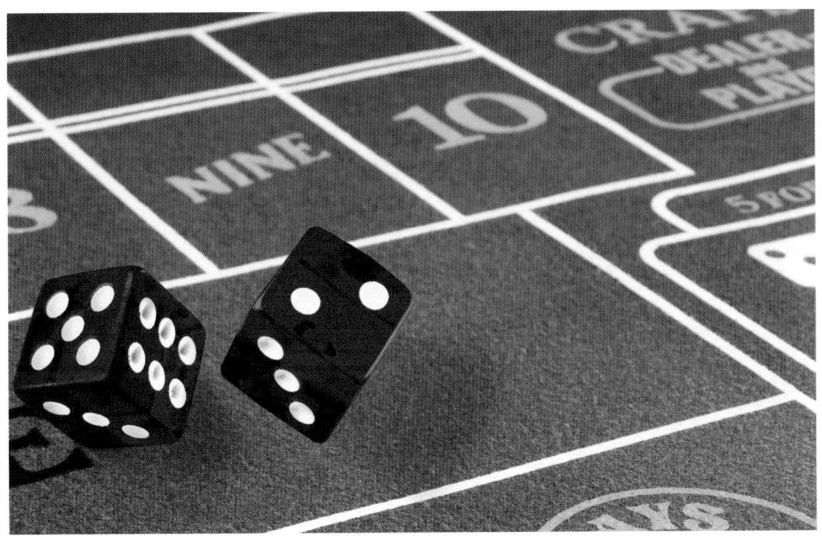

To become a better surgeon we need to understand what we mean when we talk about things like risk, odds, and probability. How can we expose our patients to a daily risk of complications and poor outcomes if we don't fully comprehend the underlying terminology?

Most people in our busy modern society are not aware that almost all significant inventions, innovations, and developments in science, economics, technology, health care, and lifestyle originated from our ability to predict future events and to make conscientious, balanced decisions on the risk and probability of our actions. The revolutionary 'risk movement' was born during the Renaissance and brought to fruition in the 16th and 17th centuries in France, Italy, and Germany by a few selected 'out of the box' pioneers. These were people who showed courage in defying the rules that had historically been defined and enforced by the church.[13]

Pragmatically speaking, the phenomenon that distinguishes our early history from modern times is the introduction of *probability theory* and *risk management*. Before the 16th century, humankind was guided by faith and belief in fate and divine intervention. It was the new mastery of risk that provided the basis for our modern society. In the 17th century, the great French mathematician and philosopher, Blaise Pascal (1623-1662), developed the first systematic method of calculating the probability of future events. (Pascal is also considered the "father of the modern theory of decision-making".)

You may have noticed how the fictitious surgeon in the preceding chapter used the terms for risk, odds, and probability interchangeably. This is likely because he just didn't know any better.

There is, of course, a difference.

By definition, *risk* is the likelihood with which a negative health outcome, complication, or adverse event will occur. It is the ratio of unfavorable outcomes compared to the total possible outcomes. In analogy, *probability* is a more generic term that relates to *any* specific outcome of interest (good or bad). The concept of *odds* is perhaps more familiar, especially to

---

[13] Bernstein PL. *Against the Gods — The Remarkable Story of Risk*. Hoboken, NJ: Wiley, 1996.

gamblers (you know who you are). Odds is defined as the ratio of the probability that a particular event will occur (e.g. a positive outcome) to the probability that it will not occur.

For example, in the game of *craps*, the *risk* (or probability) of throwing a 7 with two unbiased dice is 1:6 (i.e. 6 combinations of 36 options), whereas the *odds* of throwing a different number than a 7 are 5:1 (30 versus 6 combinations).

Probability of rolling a 7:

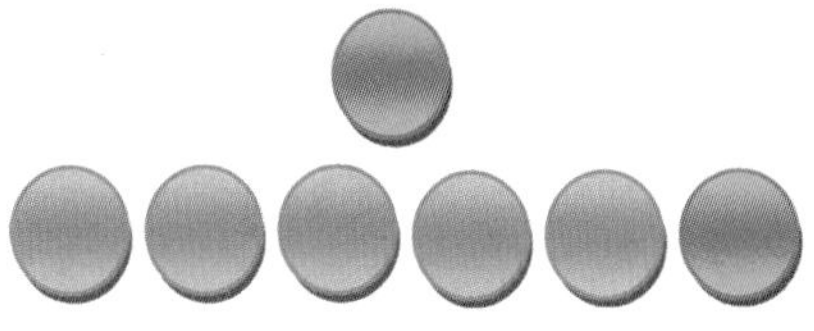

(Risk - 1:6)

Odds *against* rolling a 7:

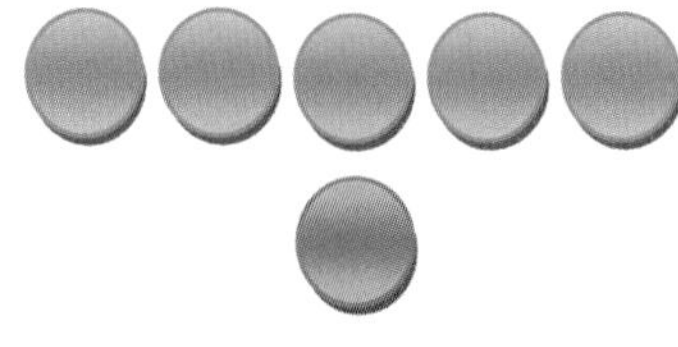

(Odds - 5:1)

Risk is typically described as a decimal number between 0 and 1, or expressed in percentages. In contrast, odds can represent a number between 0 and infinity.

A simple formula allows conversion of odds to risk and vice versa:

Risk=Odds/1+Odds
Odds=Risk/1-Risk

This is easily exemplified by a coin toss. Using an unbiased coin we get the following: the *odds* of the coin landing on heads is 1 (1:1), whereas the *probability* of heads is 0.5 (50%), and the *risk* for tails is 0.5 (50%).

The imaginary surgeon-patient interaction in the previous chapter serves to illustrate a fact I think many of us realize but don't want to admit.

Most surgeons do not understand the distinction between probability and odds and thus cannot provide coherent answers about risk, particularly in the absence of underlying valid data.

In terms of our 'Truth Test', I'm afraid the fictive surgeon has failed yet again.

Despite the obvious simplicity of the conversation, 'meet and greets' like these are a normal part of any informed consent for surgery in daily practice. In our case, the surgeon is unmasked as either ignorant or worse, dishonest. This is further aggravated by the fact that most consents are typically obtained by ancillary staff (e.g. physician assistants, interns or residents) who are frequently not qualified to understand all the technical ramifications and intricacies of a specific procedure, let alone to provide honest answers of risk estimates for complications and adverse outcomes. We've essentially delegated the 'lying' part of the informed consent to our ancillary staff.

Ouch.

In my surgical career, I've found most surgeons are quite at ease discussing the risks and odds of complications and the probability of adverse events and outcomes with patients without adequate knowledge of the terminology.

Maybe it's time for a change?

By understanding risk and probability, surgeons will be empowered to more coherently counsel their patients. Let's be clear: the ability to stratify and mitigate risk will not just keep your patients safe; this will also protect your surgical career by keeping you out of unnecessary trouble.

We'll talk about how you can minimize risk in the next chapter.

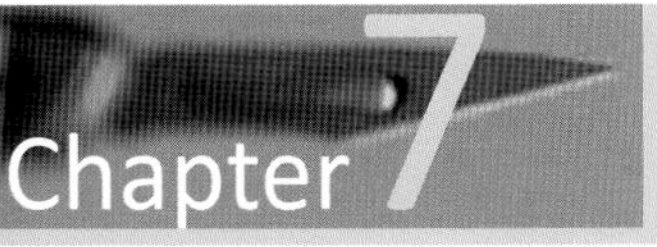

Chapter 7 Minimizing risk

"Minimizing risk is often the best we can do."
Ben Carson, MD (*1951)

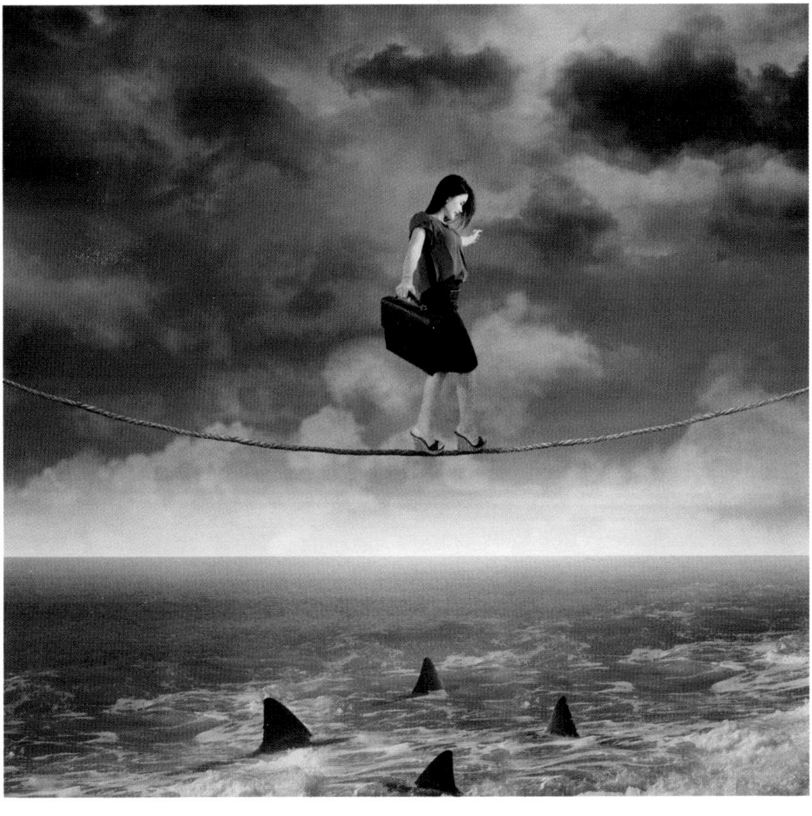

As humans, our perception of risk appears intrinsically flawed, misguided and erroneous. As a matter of fact, we tend to be alarmed and intimidated by completely irrelevant threats while underestimating the real and present dangers imposed by our daily lives. Let me elaborate on this notion by discussing a few historic anecdotes and analyzing some statistics pertinent to our 21st century society.

More than three centuries ago, Blaise Pascal coined an historic quote that is more relevant than ever to our current society and our generally unexplained and typically irrational response to threats and dangers. Pascal stated that: "Fear of harm ought to be proportional not merely to the gravity of the harm, but also to the probability of the event."

This could not be more applicable to the 21st century.

Indeed, there is widespread misperception of how odds, risk, and probability work. It is ironic that we generally feel more 'at risk' from various globally televised dangers and threats, while in truth we have literally never been any safer than we are today. Statistics published by the World Health Organization (WHO) in 2012 show an overall life expectancy of 79.8 years in the United States, 81 years in Germany and the United Kingdom, 83 years in Australia and Sweden, and an unprecedented 84.6 years in Japan! Consider that 10,000 years ago (during the Neolithic period), life expectancy at birth was just 20 years. Today, we are privileged to live more than four 'Neolithic lives'.

And guess what? Even at the beginning of the 20th century, our average life expectancy remained below 50 years.

It just doesn't add up: if we are able to live dramatically longer than ever before in history, why are we so extremely paranoid about being *less safe* and more *at risk* than during any preceding era in humankind? (the so-called "good old times").

The explanation for this massive discrepancy relates in large part to the unprecedented amount of 24/7 news coverage with non-stop exposure of horrifying events happening around the world. Recent examples include televised massacres, mass killings, and suicide bombings by militant jihadists responsible for the abduction and killing of thousands of civilians in the Middle East and in selected African countries. We are flooded with televised beheadings, burnings, and drownings of combatants and civilians by a host of radical terrorist groups whose identification and geographical location are ever changing and virtually impossible to keep track of. The territorial claim by these militant organizations is nothing less than to build a worldwide Islamic 'caliphate'.

No wonder the Western world is scared to death.

The insatiable appetite of our modern media and the recurring global travel warnings from our governments further feed the 'monster' of unjustified public intimidation and paranoia. For example, the U.S. Department of State issued a worldwide travel alert on December 19, 2014, secondary to a lone-wolf attack on a café in Sydney, Australia, that resulted in the death of two hostages.

It gets worse: on January 9, 2015, the FBI issued a worldwide caution and global travel warning, in the wake of the militant jihadist attacks at the *Charlie Hebdo* editorial office in Paris, France. The tipping point was reached in a televised interview in January 2015, when a retired CIA warfare advisor claimed that every U.S. intelligence agency had "begun to actively prepare for World War III".

Seriously?

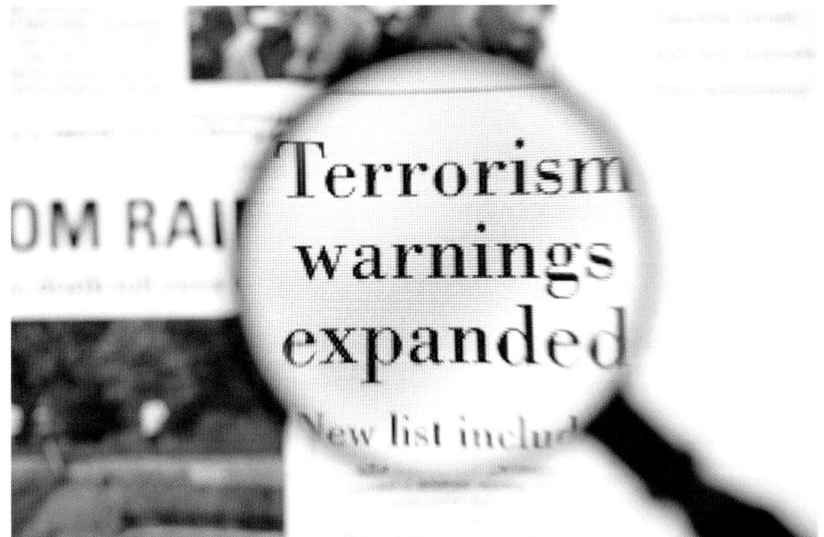

So we should stop traveling to entire continents just because there was a singular attack on a café in Australia and an *Ebola* outbreak in Africa?

Have you ever considered how enormous Africa is?

Just Google "How big is Africa compared to the United States?" and you will be astonished to see that Africa is bigger than the sum of the United States, Europe, India, Japan, and China. I'm not kidding; just check out the image below.

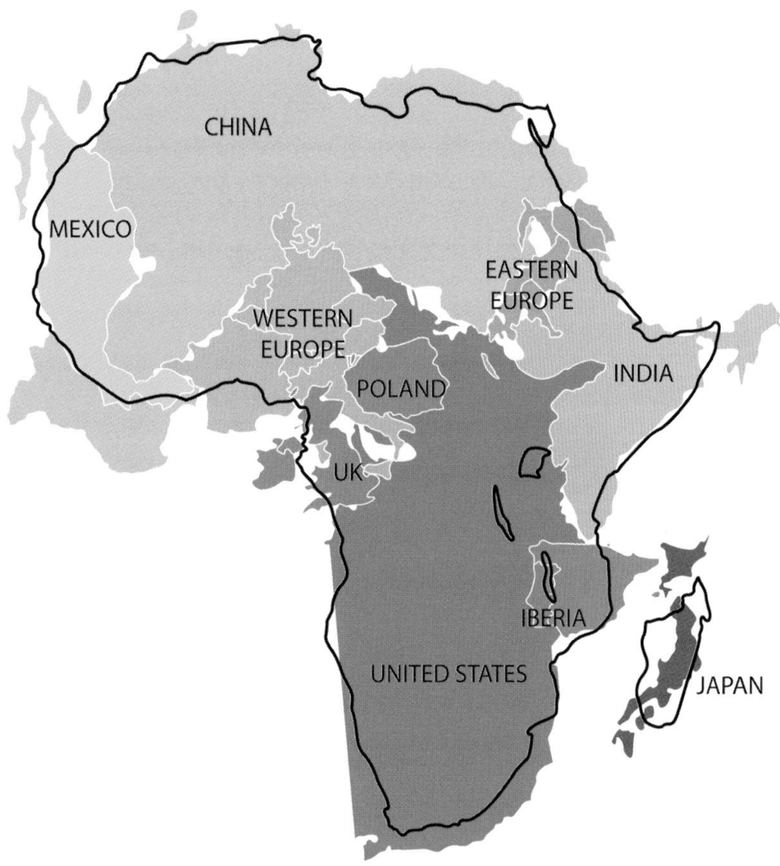

Now consider a government-issued general travel alert to Africa.

Ridiculous!

Dig this: official FBI figures show that the murder rate in Orlando is higher than in most other popular tourist destinations *outside* of the United States. Yet, this has obviously not stopped us from taking our families to Disneyworld. Nor has the State Department ever considered issuing a general travel alert to the United States.

Let's run another 'Truth Test'.

How scared should you truly be of dying from a terrorist attack?

In more than a decade since 9/11/2001, less than 40 people have been killed in terrorist attacks inside the United States (as of July 1st, 2015). Published estimates place the risk of being killed in a terrorist attack on U.S. soil at around 1:20 million. Extrapolated to your risk of dying next year, you are four times more likely to be struck by lightning (1:5 million) and 20 times more likely to drown in your own bathtub (1:1 million).

In fact, the average risk of dying at home is about 1:7,000 – the same annual risk as dying in a car crash.

Still convinced that staying at home is the safest place to be?

Former UK Prime Minister Tony Blair suitably stated in an interview in January 2015 after the *Charlie Hebdo* massacre in Paris: "Terrorists can only be successful if we feel terrorized."

Well stated.

Why don't we take a second to listen to one of the founding fathers of the United States, Benjamin Franklin, who said: "Any society that would give up a little liberty to gain a little security will deserve neither and lose both."

Seriously, what's the major killer in our Western society?

The answer is unequivocal: high blood pressure. The leading cause of cardiovascular disease, heart attacks and strokes.

Did you know that 2,200 Americans die *every day* from cardiovascular diseases? That's nearly 800,000 Americans per year, or one in every three deaths in the United States.

Shouldn't you be terrified every time you order a medium-rare filet mignon with French fries at your favorite steak house? And call security whenever the complicit Maître D' approaches your table with a salt shaker, intent on maliciously accelerating the agony of your near-certain cardiovascular death.

Let me challenge you with another brain teaser; do you know how many people fell sick or died from radiation secondary to the Fukushima Daiichi nuclear reactor accident in Japan in 2011?

The answer is *zero.*

Not a single person suffered from adverse consequences of radiation within 4 years of the nuclear disaster.

This is largely due to the fact that most of the nuclear fallout was swept out into the Pacific Ocean by eastward winds. The diluted remainder of radiation dispersed over land accumulated to an average annual exposure of 4mSv which is minimally above the Earth's background radiation of 2.4mSv.

Now dig this: around 1,600 people died from the stress of the mass evacuation from Fukushima. This includes sick and elderly people who died from heart attacks and others who committed suicide for pure fear of radiation exposure. A 4-year retrospective analysis published in *The New York Times* in 2015 stated that the Japanese government "basically panicked" and that "it was the fear of radiation that ended up killing people" — not the nuclear exposure itself.[14]

[14] Johnson G. When Radiation Isn't the Risk. *The New York Times*, Sept. 22; 2015: p.D3.

Wow!

The simple fact is that we just don't understand how to quantify and mitigate risk. We are held hostage by the common fallacy of an imaginary "quest for zero risk".

Let's face it: the risk of death in a lifetime is our only certain fate. Being paralyzed by fear and worrying alone will accomplish nothing.

The only helpful tool we have at our disposition is our ability to quantify and mitigate risk, and to make a thoughtful decision on what we consider to be a reasonable calculated risk.

Arthur Rudolph (1906-1996), a German rocket engineer during World War II who was instrumental in the development of the V-2 rocket for the Nazis and the Pershing missile and Saturn V moon rocket for NASA, stated after the first successful lunar Apollo mission in 1969:

> "You want a valve that does not leak and you try everything possible to develop one. But the real world provides you with leaky valves. You just have to determine how much leaking you can tolerate."

Let's finalize the discussion on risk mitigation by a brief focus on its relevance in medicine: current estimates suggest that more than 400,000 preventable in-hospital deaths occur in the United States every year.[15] This is roughly one sixth of all annual deaths that occur in the United States.

Obviously, the risk of dying from a medical error is dramatically higher than for any of the widely publicized hypothetical threats that are the source of our greatest fears.

The bestselling author, presidential candidate, and former Johns Hopkins neurosurgeon, Dr. Ben Carson, provides a pragmatic and practicable approach to decision making in the face of an uncertain

[15] James JT. A new evidence-based estimate of patient harms associated with hospital care. *Journal of Patient Safety* 2013; 9: 122-8.

outcome. In his outstanding book, *Take the Risk*,[16] Ben Carson suggests four questions to help determine when to take a calculated risk:

- "What is the *best* thing that can happen if I take the risk?"
- "What is the *worst* thing that can happen if I take the risk?"
- "What is the *best* thing that can happen if I don't take the risk?"
- "What is the *worst* thing that can happen if I don't take the risk?"

Simple and pragmatic.

I've personally applied this approach for risk stratification in my own practice for many years now. You should try it, too! This decision-making exercise will help you stay out of trouble and will eventually save some of your patients' lives.

Let me finalize this discussion with a philosophical call to enjoy life independent of perceived risk, by citing my favorite quote from the American journalist and author, Hunter S. Thompson (1937-2005):

> "Life should not be a journey to the grave with the intention of arriving safely in a pretty and well preserved body, but rather to skid in broadside in a cloud of smoke, thoroughly used up, totally worn out, and loudly proclaiming: Wow! What a ride!"

[16] Carson B. *Take the Risk*. Grand Rapids, MI: Zondervan, 2008.

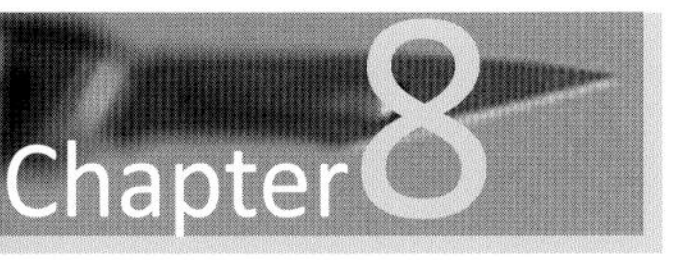

How to deal with uncertainty

"The only man who never makes a mistake is the man who never makes a decision."

Theodore Roosevelt (1858-1919)

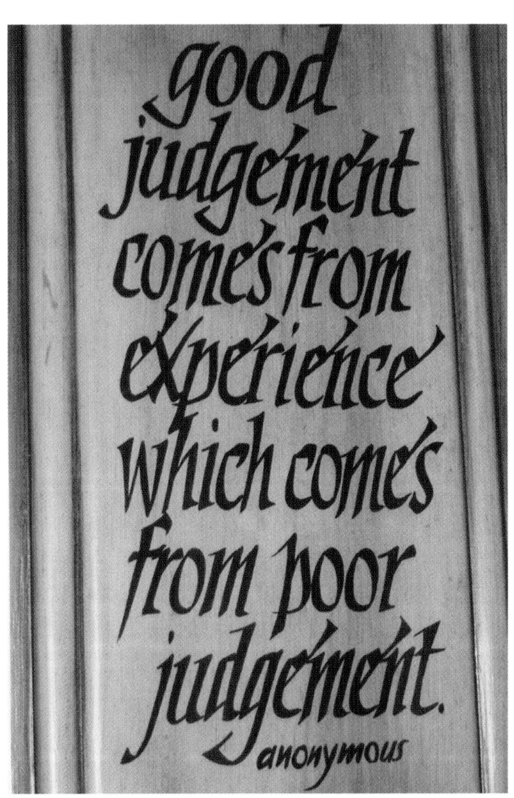

One of the hardest parts of being a surgeon is our level of uncertainty. No matter how much we read and learn over the years, how extensively we train and practice, we have to live with a sizeable amount of uncertainty.

For example, I recently performed a complex spine fusion in a patient who broke his neck after slipping and falling in his hotel room. I placed eight screws around his cervical spine and took the pressure off his spinal cord. Quite a standard procedure.

Yet, before closing the wound, I felt that one screw just didn't look quite right on the final intra-operative radiographs. I scrutinized all kinds of different dedicated fluoroscopy views, and still was not certain that the screw was correct. I then simply followed one of my own decision-making algorithms that I had established over the years: if I question the position of a screw for more than 5 minutes, I will exchange the screw. Good thing I did. That particular screw was too close to the spinal cord and needed to be changed. No harm to the patient. Just another one of those mentally draining and fatiguing decision-making processes. I'm glad I made a good call on this one. But how many times am I wrong? How many times do I settle for compromise and potentially poor decisions, either because I just don't know any better or out of pure complacency? This phenomenon is called "decision fatigue".

There's a solution to the problem, however. A concept called the "expected utility theory". If you're not familiar with it, that's probably because it's something that isn't taught in medical school.

The concept itself is pragmatic and straightforward: it's designed as a way to help you rationally determine an outcome of an action with uncertain consequences by helping you choose the highest expected "utility". In other words, it directs you towards the action with the highest likelihood of a positive patient outcome in the face of uncertainty. Just as I did by applying my internal algorithm of automatically changing a screw around the spine if I spend more than 5 minutes questioning whether I should.

There are many additional sources of poor judgment and errors in human reasoning. Let me entertain you with a few of those. In the preceding two chapters, we became experts in understanding risk and probability. Well, let me ask you if you've heard about the concept of "conditional probability"?

Are you thinking that this is getting way too theoretical and irrelevant for the care of your patients? You're saying to yourself, maybe I should just skip to the next chapter? Or put the book away altogether?

Well, hold your horses, and let me challenge you with a clinical scenario.

Let's pretend that you're a patient and you've just dragged yourself into your primary care physician's office. You feel sick. You show up at your doc's office with a fever of 103°F (39.4°C). You're shivering. You're worried. Lately, the press has gone nuts with in-depth 24/7 coverage of a

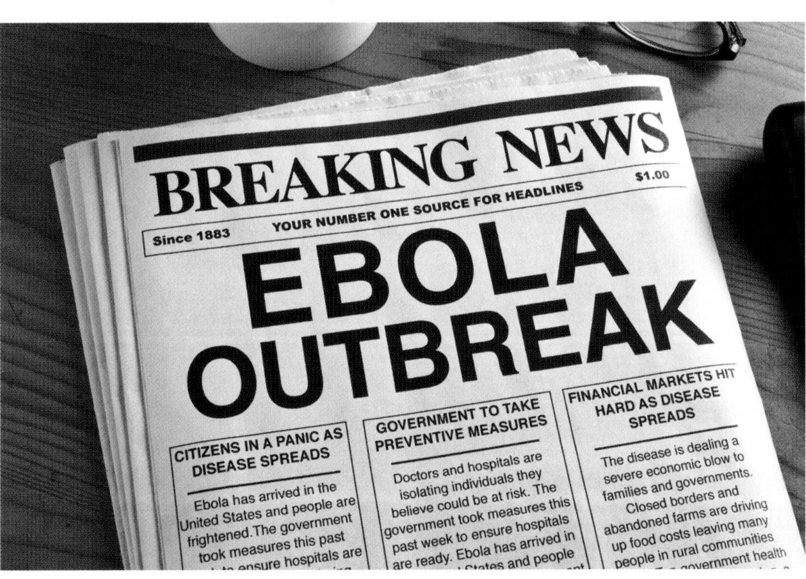

horrific and widespread outbreak of *Ebola* in West Africa. You want to make sure you don't have the deadly hemorrhagic fever.

Given that you are freaking out, the doctor offers to run a new rapid *Ebola* screening test that has a 99% sensitivity and 99% specificity. In other words, this test will show that you either do or do not have the disease with 99% certainty. So you give a blood sample and wait anxiously in the office for the results, knees knocking on the edge of the examining table. When your doc ambles back into the room and tells you that your *Ebola* test turned out positive, you want to run out screaming and commit suicide. Hang on! Don't lose your cool just yet. What's the actual probability that you truly have the disease?

Could it be 99%?

Is it more like 50% (the same as flipping a coin)?

Maybe it's as low as 1%?

Or in an imaginary 'best case', could it be less than 0.001%?

I often use this exact scenario as a trivia challenge to my colleagues at the hospital and at social gatherings with friends and family (I've always been a trivia guy).

What's striking is that I invariably get the same answer:

"Well, if the test is 99% sensitive and 99% specific, that means that I have *Ebola* with 99% certainty!"

Do you want to revise your answer, or is it final? I ask.

Absolutely final. 99% certain.

Is that the answer you'd give your patients as well?

Really?

You're as wrong as you can be, because you didn't take into account the law of conditional probability.

Here's the correct answer: statistically, your risk of being infected with *Ebola* is less than 0.0001%!

Seriously, it's that low despite your doc's 99% sensitive test.

Bottom line: you don't have *Ebola*.

The logic here is simple, actually. Conditional probability is based on Bayes' Theorem.

Thomas Bayes (1701-1761) was an English minister and statistician who figured this out 250 years ago. His groundbreaking theory still allows us to predict tomorrow's weather and to provide a high level of certainty to a clinical diagnosis.

There you go: a practical solution for the surgeon's residual uncertainty!

In essence, Bayes' Theorem allows us to predict a probability (P) of an event (A) that occurs in dependence of a previous event (B), according to the formula:

$$P(A \backslash B) = \frac{P(B \backslash A)\ P(A)}{P(B)}$$

Remember you were freaking out at the doc's office? Let's apply Bayes' Theorem to your request for a rapid *Ebola* test.

In 2014, there were four confirmed cases of *Ebola* virus infections in the United States (and only one of these patients died). Based on an estimated U.S. population of 318 million (2014), the prevalence of *Ebola* in the United States was much less than one in a million.

Thus, even with a highly sensitive test that catches 99% of all true positive patients, the number of false-positive test results (1%) will still massively outnumber those very few people who truly have the disease.

Even if we overestimate the number of *Ebola*-infected patients in the United States to be 100 patients in 300 million, 99 patients will have a correct diagnosis (99% true positives), whereas 2,999,999 patients of the remaining 299,999,900 healthy subjects will be wrongly diagnosed (1% false positives).

Thus, the likelihood of having *Ebola* in the presence of a positive test is 99/(99+2,999,999). That is just about 0.00003% (with four trailing zeroes). It's kind of a big deal to be able to tell your patient who just got horrified about a new deadly diagnosis that, despite the test being positive, he or she does not have the disease.

Are you a believer now?

We as surgeons have come a long way in successfully masking uncertainty. Our professors in medical school and residency trained us to practice with dogmatic certainty. The more we specialize in our postgraduate training, the more we get comfortable with a false sense of certainty, based on the premise: "that's how we've always done it." Once we've practiced long enough, we eventually consider ourselves 'experts' in a specific field. This basically means that our level of erroneous certainty is now irrevocably cast in stone.

Let's be honest: most of the stuff we do in surgery is eventually made up. Over time, the empirical practice taught through generations turns into an unquestioned standard of care. "We'll do it this way because the 'expert' says so!"

And who would dare to question an over-specialized expert in a certain medical field? In all these years of practicing as an academic surgeon, I've traveled around the world to give invited lectures, from South America to Europe, to the Middle East, India, and Hong Kong. And in all these years, I've invariably felt that the community labeling me an expert was unjustified. This notion is nicely summarized by Wade Smith, my close friend of many years and esteemed surgeon colleague in Denver, who provided the following spot-on definition: "An expert is someone from out of town with slides."

Maybe you'd guess that the modern age of evidence-based medicine (EBM) will finally extinguish our residual level of clinical uncertainty?

Seriously?!

Don't get me started.

Have you ever heard of the "garbage in — garbage out" paradigm for flawed interpretations of the published literature? Have you ever taken into consideration that evidence-based best practices may pose a huge ethical dilemma to the surgeon scientist and have a negative downstream effect on the development of new innovative strategies to treat our patients?

For example, if an evidence-based guideline tells you to treat all of your patients suffering from acute spinal cord injuries with high-dose steroids, you're really screwed if: 1) you opt out of this established "standard of care" (how do you explain this to the judge?); or 2) you attempt to design a new trial to prove the ineffectiveness of steroids, as your institutional review board won't approve your research project due to the ethical concern of depriving the control patients of a proven "evidence-based" treatment option.

Let's jump on this example of a historic disaster where evidence-based medicine possibly killed hundreds or thousands of patients.

In the 1980s, the multi-center double-blind randomized controlled NASCIS trials proclaimed that the early application of high-dose steroids (methylprednisolone) was an efficacious pharmacologic therapy for patients suffering from acute spinal cord injury.[17]

These recommendations were subsequently considered an evidence-based best practice (so-called "level 1" evidence) and faithfully adhered to around the globe for almost two decades.

[17] Bracken MB, *et al.* A randomized, controlled trial of methylprednisolone or naloxone in the treatment of acute spinal-cord injury. Results of the Second National Acute Spinal Cord Injury Study. *New England Journal of Medicine* 1990; 322: 1405-11.

If it was not for a bright, independent 'out-of-the-box' thinker, Dr. R. John Hurlbert, a neurosurgeon from the University of Calgary Spine Program in Canada, we would still be harming and killing our patients by the *Trojan Horse* of high-dose steroids.

In the late 1990s, Dr. Hurlbert critically questioned the value of steroids by considering the potential harm induced to the patients under his care. He actually took the time and diligence to perform a so-called "post-hoc analysis" of the entire raw data set from the original NASCIS trials.[18] Dr. Hurlbert's analysis single-handedly revealed that the postulated efficacy of methylprednisolone had in fact been due to pure chance, and that the underlying raw data failed to prove a relevant improvement in neurological paralysis after spinal cord injury.

Ironically, Dr. Hurlbert's revelations (and provocative publications) were largely ridiculed in the surgical community. It wasn't until the dramatic failure of the multicenter prospective randomized CRASH trial on more than 10,000 patients that Dr. Hurlbert's hypothesis was proven once and for all. The study finally revealed that high-dose steroids are harmful (instead of beneficial) for patients with neurological injuries.[19]

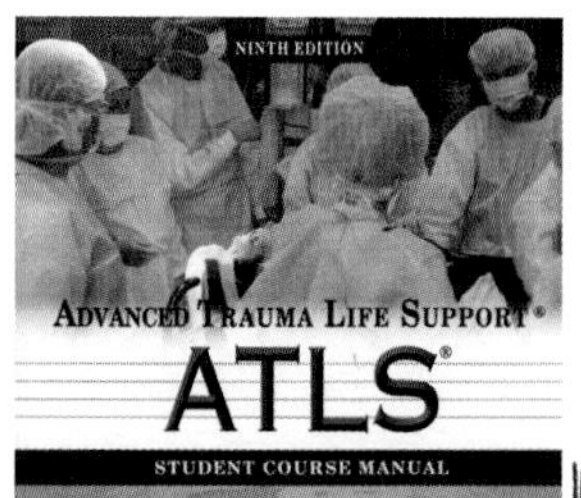

GENERAL MANAGEMENT 191

not improve after a fluid challenge, the judicious use of vasopressors may be indicated. Phenylephrine hydrochloride, dopamine, or norepinephrine is recommended. Overzealous fluid administration may cause pulmonary edema in patients with neurogenic shock. When the fluid status is uncertain, the use of invasive monitoring may be helpful. A urinary catheter is inserted to monitor urinary output and prevent bladder distention.

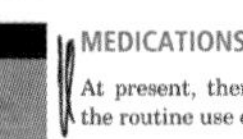

MEDICATIONS

At present, there is insufficient evidence to support the routine use of steroids in spinal cord injury.

TRANSFER

Patients with spine fractures or neurologic deficit should be transferred to a definitive-care facility. The safest procedure is to transfer the patient after telephone consultation with a spine specialist. Avoid unnecessary delay. Stabilize the patient and apply the necessary splints, backboard, and/or semirigid cervical collar. **Remember, cervical spine injuries above C6 can result in partial or total loss of respiratory function.** If there is any concern about the adequacy of ventilation, the patient should be intubated prior to transfer.

Scenario ■ conclusion The patient was admitted to the intensive care unit, underwent fixation of his cervical spine, and was ultimately transferred to a spinal cord rehabilitation center.

Advanced Trauma Life Support® (ATLS®) guideline for the use of steroids in patients with spinal cord injuries, 9th edition, 2012. Reprinted with permission. © American College of Surgeons.

---

18 Hurlbert RJ. Methylprednisolone for acute spinal cord injury: an inappropriate standard of care. *Journal of Neurosurgery* 2000; 93: 1-7.

19 Sauerland S, Maegele M. A CRASH landing in severe head injury. *The Lancet* 2004; 364: 1291-2.

The subsequent global reversal in practice was preceded by nearly two decades of uncritical administration of a ‘deadly drug’ to a highly vulnerable patient population under the umbrella of an evidence-based standard of care.

Are you still with me?

Still unquestionably dedicated to evidence-based medicine as the *Holy Grail* for medical decision-making?

If so, I have more cool stuff to share with you.

Have you heard of “publication bias”? This is another hidden flaw and unrecognized source of error in published meta-analyses and clinical guidelines.

Publication bias is introduced by the preferred selection of published articles that provide positive and statistically significant results over those with negative findings.

Let me drop another story on you. When I started working as an orthopaedic trauma surgeon at Denver Health in 2006, I made the coincidental acquaintance of a Swiss fellow surgeon, Erik Hasenboehler, who had just lost a job opportunity at a busy trauma center in Houston, Texas.

Stranded in Denver, Erik inquired about performing research under my mentorship. In an attempt to keep him busy, I encouraged Erik to address a question that had been on my mind for a long time: how many surgical papers publish negative results?

Poor Erik. If he only saw this coming, he would have immediately reimmigrated back to Switzerland. I tasked him with a huge endeavor: to run a study screening more than 30,000 articles published in a dozen representative and prestigious journals in the field of surgery and orthopaedics (see Table 1).

Table 1. Overview on the 12 selected peer-reviewed journals analyzed in our study. Journal ranking[1] and journal impact factors[2] were retrieved from the Institute for Scientific Information (ISI) database from 2006. Journal ranking was determined by the specific subject categories of Surgery* and Orthopedics§. The numbers of articles analyzed in this study are shown as the overall publications[3] (including non-original articles) and as original articles exclusively.[4] Articles were assessed in all individual journals' volumes from January 2000 until December 2006. Reprinted with permission from: Hasenboehler E, *et al.* Bias towards publishing positive results in orthopedic and general surgery: a patient safety issue? *Patient Saf Surg* 2007; 1: 4. (Creative Commons Attribution License, BioMed Central Ltd.)

Journal title	Journal ranking[1]	Impact factor[2]	Total number of articles analyzed[3]	Number of original papers analyzed[4]
Annals of Surgery	1*	7.678	1,835	1,277
Journal of Bone and Joint Surgery (American)	4§	2.444	3,012	1,501
British Journal of Surgery	5*	4.092	2,607	1,258
Spine	5§	2.351	4,357	2,860
Journal of Bone and Joint Surgery (British)	11§	1.790	2,364	1,415
Journal of Orthopaedic Trauma	13§	1.670	1,270	494
Archives of Surgery	14*	3.058	2,254	1,026
Surgery	15*	2.977	2,714	1,404
Journal of the American College of Surgeons	16*	2.813	2,437	866
Journal of Trauma	38*	2.035	3,316	1,979
World Journal of Surgery	45*	1.765	2,144	1,326
Injury	76*	1.067	1,887	991
All journals			**30,197**	**16,397**

My hypothesis was that my own favorite journals published more positive and statistically relevant data than negative results.

Oh boy, was I right.

After 6 months of impeccable work, endless commitment and dedication (and close to resignation!), Erik presented me with his findings: 74% of all screened articles presented positive data, 17% published negative (yet statistically significant) results, and only 9% of all articles were neutral.

You say: "So what?"

I say: this is a huge deal!

Clearly, our 'best practice' clinical guidelines rely on the full body of available published data. Withholding knowledge from failed trials and from negative studies that show *no effect* of a specific treatment will give us the false (yet statistically significant) confidence that we are treating our patients with the best available quality care, when in truth doing the opposite (or nothing at all) may be more efficacious and safer!

Get it?

By the way, the globally renowned scientific 'guerilla' consortium *The Edge* (consisting of multiple Nobel laureates and other renowned forefront thinkers and scientists) recently recommended to completely abolish evidence-based medicine as an outdated tenet.[20]

Are you still convinced that evidence-based medicine resolves our ultimate level of uncertainty?

Maybe not, huh?!

In essence, there are three types of uncertainties:

- *Type 1* uncertainty reflects incomplete or imperfect individual knowledge of all the available science and published literature; this

[20] www.edge.org/annual-questions.

basically implies that we "didn't do our homework" if we don't know it.

- *Type 2* uncertainty mirrors the shortcomings of evidence-based medicine discussed above; this reflects all the unanswered questions in medicine, independent of our individual knowledge. We can't know it even if we read all the published papers in the world.
- *Type 3* uncertainty is a combination of the two entities described above; this is when we are unable to distinguish whether we are simply ignorant (or lazy), or whether the clinical question truly remains unanswered within the vast body of the current medical knowledge.

Test yourself: anytime you're uncertain about making a medical decision, attempt to classify your level of uncertainty. You'll be surprised to see how many times you get stuck in type 2 uncertainty, where an unequivocal standard of care just does not exist, in light of the paucity of data and poor quality studies performed in a specific field.

Whatever you take back to your practice from this bulk of information, just do me one favor: don't follow published EBM guidelines blindly. Those clearly don't replace your residual level of uncertainty.

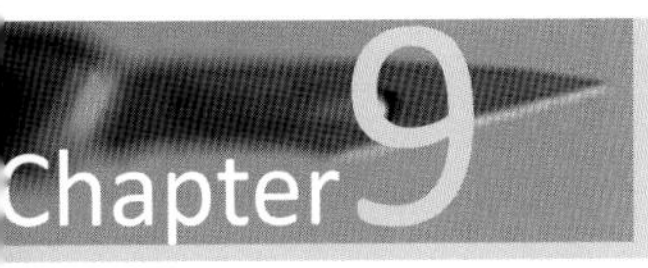

Chapter 9 You can't fix what you don't know!

"I do my best to avoid difficulties and any kind of complications. I like everything around me to be clear as crystal."

Alfred Hitchcock (1899-1980)

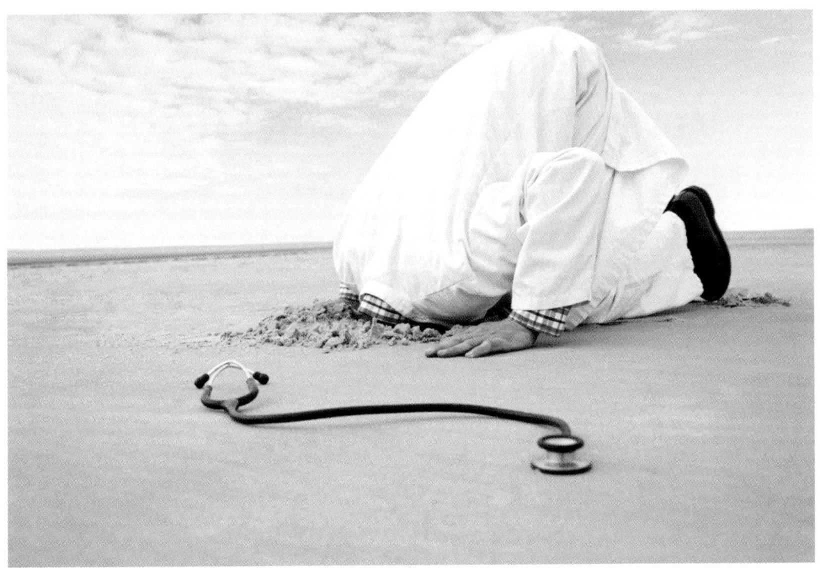

Let's face it — despite the overwhelming amount of risk, unknown probabilities, and residual uncertainty, there is one single aspect of our surgical practice over which we have full control: we can choose to know our own complication rate.

And guess what? Most of us don't!

As emphasized in the fictive case scenario from Chapter 5, we either make up our numbers with an imaginary "1% to 2%" expected complication rate, or we dramatically understate all the stuff that goes wrong every day.

The fictitious surgeon from the earlier chapter eroded his professional credibility by using interchangeably the distinct terms "surgical complication", "adverse event", "postoperative infection" and "outcome". It's worth noting that the postoperative infection rate is, by definition, just a subset of the overall complication rate, which again represents a subset of the overall "adverse event" rate (see the graph below).

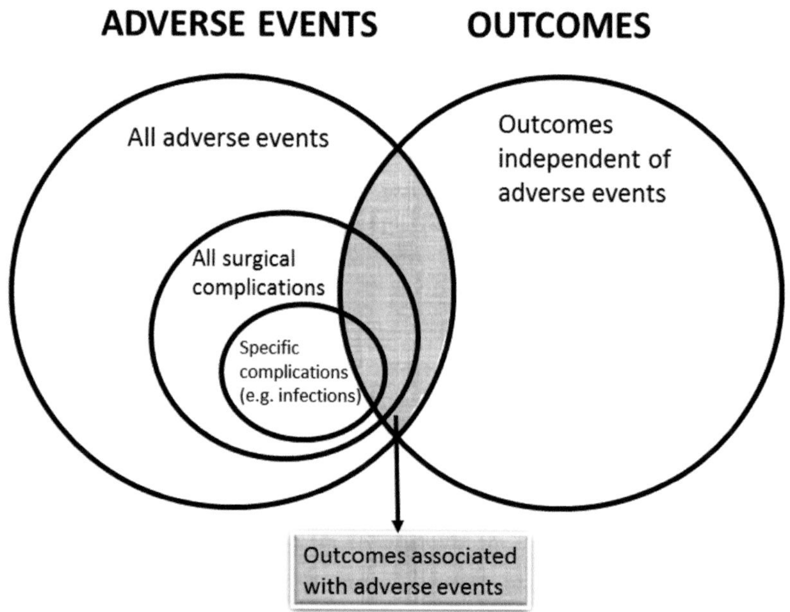

In contrast, an "outcome" is a different entity. For example, a patient may sustain an adverse event or a complication and nevertheless show an excellent overall outcome. This is exemplified by the case of a postoperative superficial wound infection that is successfully managed by a few days of oral antibiotics, without any long-term consequences. In contrast, another patient whose surgical procedure was impeccable and short-term recovery uneventful may suffer from a poor long-term outcome. The latter example is illustrated by a patient undergoing a spinal fusion surgery for chronic lower back pain. While the objective results may be excellent, with the absence of any intra-operative complications, pristine wound healing, stellar postoperative radiographs and achieved CT-proven spine fusion over time, this patient may still continue suffering from chronic refractory back pain despite the risky invasive procedure having been performed per state-of-the-art.

Thus, subjective outcomes may not correlate with objective quality and safety metrics associated with a specific surgical procedure.

Makes sense, right?

As surgeons, we're actually quite proficient at neglecting our own shortcomings and complications in a very cavalier fashion. We have an entire career at our disposal to practice suppressing our own failures by putting our head in the sand about all the problems we create for our patients.

How would you react if the technician of the nuclear power plant in your community decided to be as sloppy in recognition and mitigation of adverse occurrences as we deal with our own complication rates?

Let me make a bold request:

Under the premise that "You can't fix what you don't know!" it is our obligation as surgeons and stewards of arguably the most prestigious and rewarding profession on this planet, to diligently scrutinize, report, review and disclose all complications that occur on our watch in a standardized and proactive fashion. How can we possibly become better surgeons tomorrow if we don't recognize and mitigate our shortcomings of today?

You think we can't do any better, and we're doing our best?

Let me challenge you with a success story from our own department: data from our Quality Improvement (QI) initiative at Denver Health show a dramatic increase in our orthopedic group's complication rate by nearly *five-fold* during a 6-year window from 2004 to 2009.

How is this a success story? Sounds more like an example of dramatic failure? Are we just getting sloppier as we get older?

Or did we possibly become more honest and diligent in recognizing, analyzing and reporting our own complications? If so, how did that happen?

When I joined Denver Health in 2006, the format of the so-called "M&M" (Morbidity & Mortality) conferences was at the discretion of individual department leadership, and not mandated in a standardized fashion. Back then, our QI process relied on the pure voluntary reporting of occasional surgical complications by individual surgeons. These selected 'worst case' complications were then presented by the most junior members of the team (interns and second-year residents) at an M&M 'horror show' that occurred every other month.

Those case presentations focused exclusively on horrible scenarios when patients had bled to death, died on the OR table from acute pulmonary embolism, or had their wrong leg cut off accidentally. While the 'thrill-seeking' aspect of such a filtered process is unquestionable, its educational opportunity remains limited by under-reporting of complications. Furthermore, this selective approach doesn't give consideration to instances when things almost went wrong, but did not reach the patient (*near misses*), or when errors reached the patient but coincidentally did not cause any harm (*no harm events*).

At the time, our residents in training were rightfully hesitant to report complications. Their willingness to speak up would immediately be punished by the subsequent task of creating a lengthy PowerPoint lecture, presenting the case and taking the heat of being 'pimped' by the senior surgeons in the audience for complications that were obviously not even created by the presenter.

The system was wrong, so it had to be fixed.

In a team approach, we completely redesigned our departmental QI process in 2007 based on the principles outlined in Table 2.

Table 2. Rules of engagement in our orthopedic QI process at Denver Health.

- Any member of the team is fully entitled to anonymously report any suspected adverse occurrence in "real time" (i.e. surgeons, residents, nurses, students).
- Occurrences are reported to an independent nurse provider in charge of managing the departmental adverse-event database.
- A "no fault" policy for reporting occurrences is encouraged with strong support from the departmental leadership.
- Peer review of each reported event occurs at a departmental M&M conference once a week (Monday mornings). All reported events from the preceding week are discussed and reviewed using a standardized case review form (see the figure overleaf).
- Case reviews are exclusively performed in the presence of the responsible attending surgeon, the involved residents in training, and at least two additional faculty staff members who were not involved in the occurrence.
- A corrective action is defined for each reviewed case, as deemed necessary for resolution of the problem and prevention of a similar occurrence in the future.
- There are no punitive measures against the reporter, the involved surgeon, and the members of the care team.
- Each closed case is prospectively entered into a departmental QI database.
- All team members involved in the adverse occurrence are notified about the final assessment of the review process.

Name: **Admitted:**

Ortho M&M: **Ortho Team:** /

MRN: **FIN:** **Trauma #:**

Reported Event:

I. Status

- ☐ A. Complication
- ☐ B. "Near miss" event
- ☐ C. "No harm" event
- ☐ D. Death
- ☐ E. Not a complication
- ☐ F. Not an Ortho complication

II. Specific Complication

- ☐ A. Postoperative infection
- ☐ B. Failure of reduction/fixation
- ☐ C. Misplaced implant
- ☐ D. Fracture-Nonunion
- ☐ E. Wound healing issue
- ☐ F. Failure of flap or replantation
- ☐ G. Postop bleeding/hematoma
- ☐ H. Vascular injury
- ☐ I. Neurologic injury
- ☐ J. Medical complication
- ☐ K. DVT/PE
- ☐ L. Death
- ☐ M. Other: ____________________
- ☐ N. Missed Injury

III. Patient Harm

1. DHMCQSS

- ☐ QSS 1: "No harm" to patient
- ☐ QSS 2: "No harm", but increased risk of harm
- ☐ QSS 3: Harm requiring escalation of care
- ☐ QSS 4: Harm resulting in prolonged disability
- ☐ QSS 5: Life threatening or resulting in death

2. Revision Surgery

- ☐ None
- ☐ Yes - Planned Return to OR
- ☐ Yes - Unplanned return to OR

IV. Contributing Root Cause

- ☐ A. Communication
- ☐ B. Supervision
- ☐ C. Indication
- ☐ D. Technique
- ☐ E. Treatment concept
- ☐ F. Judgment error
- ☐ G. Aftercare
- ☐ H. System issue

(A–H: Preventable VI. - 1)

- ☐ I. Patient compliance
- ☐ J. Patient selection
- ☐ K. Co-morbidities
- ☐ L. Injury severity

(I–L: Non-Preventable VI. - 3)

- ☐ M. No root cause evident — Equivocal VI. - 4
- ☐ N. Other: ____________________

V. Corrective Action

- ☐ A. Education at QA Conference
- ☐ B. Guideline/protocol
- ☐ C. To PI Committee/Peer Review

VI. Preventability

- ☐ 1. Preventable
- ☐ 2. Potentially Preventable
- ☐ 3. Non-Preventable
- ☐ 4. Equivocal

- ☐ A. Disease Related
- ☐ B. Provider-Related
- ☐ C. System-Related

VII. Disclosure

- ☐ A. Occurred
- ☐ B. Did not occur - Reason: ____________________

____

Procedure Start: **Heparin Start:**

Procedure End:

Antibiotics Start: **Last Heparin:**

Total Tourniquet Time:

Loop Closure Comments:

- ☐ No deviation from standard of care
- ☐ See separate dictation
- ☐ Deferred loop closure to PI Committee

Definitions:

Complication: Any event that deviates from an anticipated uneventful recovery from illness or surgery

"Near Miss" Event: An unplanned event with the potential of resulting in a preventable injury, which was recognized and aborted in time before inducing patient harm.

"No Harm" Event: An unplanned event which was not recognized or aborted in time, but did not result in patient harm, and did not meet the criteria for the definition of a "true" complication.

Unplanned Return to OR: Any return to the OR for an unanticipated event or complication

Preventable: Expected or unexpected sequela of procedure, disease or injury that is likely to have been prevented or substantially ameliorated by taking appropriate steps.

Non-Preventable: Expected or unexpected sequela for which reasonable and appropriate preventive steps had been taken

Potentially Preventable: Expected or unexpected sequela which had the potential to be prevented or substantially ameliorated.

Confidential Privileged Quality Management Documenper C.R.S. § 25-3-109

M&M case review form (version 2014) for weekly peer review of all reported adverse events and suspected complications at the Department of Orthopedic Surgery at Denver Health.

Guess what? It worked. It was unbelievable.

The entire team bought in and participated. Surgeons started voluntarily reporting their own complications (unheard of!).

By 2010, we performed a first retrospective analysis of our QI database to compare reports before and after implementation of the new M&M process.[21] The analysis spanned 3 years before to 3 years after implementation of our new initiative.

The number of surgical procedures performed during both time windows was in a similar range (n=6,191 vs. n=6,845). The relative number of reported occurrences was stratified by those individual surgeons who participated during both time periods. Surgeons who were previously reluctant to report their own complications increased the reporting of suspected adverse events from the 'magic' number of 1%-2% (2004-2006) to more than 12% (2007-2010) of all surgical cases. Some reports were even reviewed as "not a complication" — a strong surrogate marker for open reporting and over-screening of occurrences.

The aggregate percentage of occurrences determined to be true complications after the weekly peer-review process increased from 1.4% to 6.7% (see the figure overleaf).

And herein lies the paradox: as our group of surgeons gained experience and surgical skills over nearly 6 years, our surgical complication rate increased by *five-fold*. But, more impressively, our group was able to establish a new culture of reporting that was embraced by the entire team, thanks to the new open-minded and non-punitive system.

I'm sure we'd all rather be operated on by an honest surgeon who transparently admits that his true complication rate is 6.7% than by a surgeon who is oblivious of his failures and claims a complication rate of "around 1% to 2%".

Right?

---

[21] Stahel PF, *et al.* Disclosure and reporting of surgical complications - a double-edged sword? *American Journal of Medical Quality* 2010; 25: 398-402.

Obviously, you would need to explain to your patients why honestly reported statistics look different than the generic (made-up) estimates by less critical surgeons.

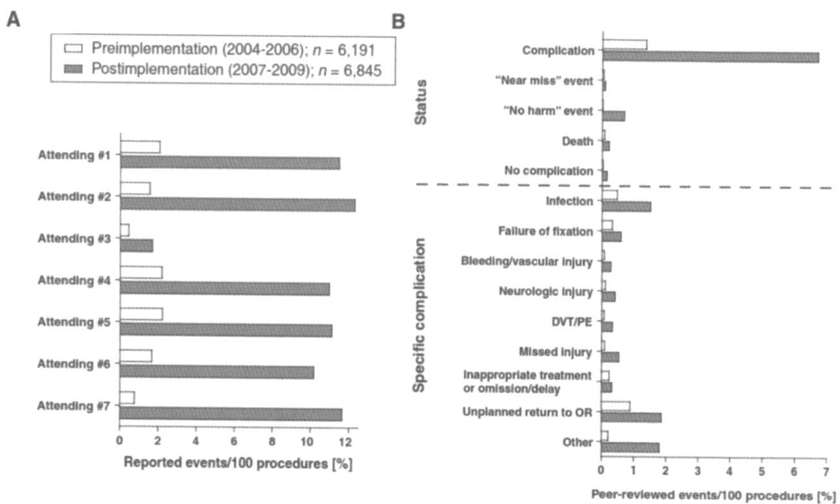

Reported events per attending surgeon, shown as percentages (number of events per 100 surgical procedures), during the pre-implementation and post-implementation phases of the new QA process (A) and grading of occurrences after weekly peer review, shown as occurrences per 100 surgical procedures for the entire department (B). Abbreviations: QA = quality assurance; DVT = deep venous thrombosis; PE = pulmonary embolism; OR = operating room. Reprinted with permission from: Stahel PF, *et al.* Disclosure and reporting of surgical complications - a double-edged sword? *Am J Med Qual* 2010; 25: 398-402. © SAGE Publications Inc.

The next step in becoming a better surgeon is to know and understand the detailed underlying data related to our surgical performance, including all the 'bad stuff' that happens on our watch.

As for any other high-risk industry, this expanded knowledge gives us the ability to fix problems that we are currently not even aware exist at all.

Chapter 10 Individual accountability

"I never make exceptions. An exception disproves the rule."

Sherlock Holmes, in Sir Arthur Conan Doyle's *The Sign of Four* (1890)

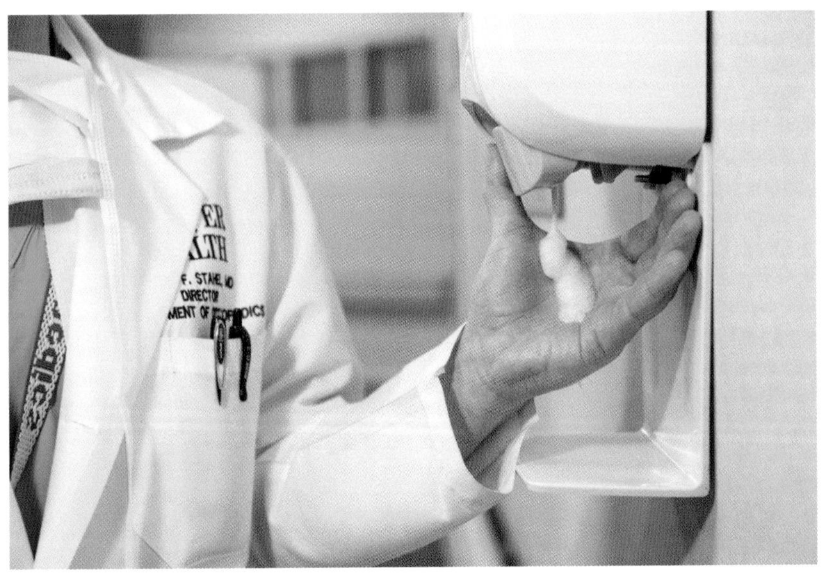

I'll be the first to admit all this information can be overwhelming.

Maybe even a bit annoying.

I've gone from emotional anecdotes from my own failures to lecturing you on logic, stats, and numbers. You're most likely thinking that everything we've talked about, the intricacies of life as a surgeon, is so complex and unpredictable that it's largely out of your own control.

What's the good of all this information if it doesn't mean a damn when the "chips are down"?

I told you that being empathetic is imperative for being a better surgeon, yet, I was unable to give you a scientifically accurate working definition of empathy. Then I had the nerve to suggest some 'Truth Tests', rammed some formulae down your throat, and bored you with the theory on risk and probability (all of which, you could argue, may be of interest to a seventh grader at best). Worse, I risked being perceived as dogmatic and condescending when I insinuated that you don't listen to your patients and that you may not have the faintest idea about your own complication rate. Then, just to hammer home my intrinsic addiction to conflict and debate, I even dared to question the value of evidence-based medicine as a 'safe haven' to guide the standard of care in your practice.

I did all of that and provided you with very little in the way of practical advice.

No tools. No checklists. No hands-on 'tips and tricks'.

I'm certainly not trying to waste your time. I'm trying to open your eyes. The truth is: you're reading this far into the book because you want to be a better, safer, more effective surgeon. In my mind, putting empathetic care into practice is just like any elevating endeavor — you have to know where you're coming from and be willing to change.

With that out of the way, here's my simple and pragmatic 'manifesto' on becoming a better surgeon, based on three solid pillars:

- Personal accountability.
- Credible leadership 'in the trenches'.
- Role modeling without excuses or exceptions.

In other words, walk the walk, don't just talk the talk.

Sounds very generic, and maybe too trivial, right?

From my years of experience, I am personally convinced that, put in practice, these three basic concepts keep our patients safe. When we serve as role models and hold our team and trainees accountable for their actions at all times, we win. All of us win — patients and surgeons.

As Winston Churchill said in his landmark 'finest hour' speech to the House of Commons after the evacuation from Dunkirk on June 4, 1940: "Every morning brought forth a noble chance, and every chance brought forth a noble knight." Churchill then concluded his speech with the simple imperative: "We shall never surrender!"

To bring his words into our profession, as 'surgical healers' we are charged to uphold patient safety to its highest standards. We shall be the noble knights fighting for our patients. We shall never compromise the safety of our patients. We shall never make or take excuses, or tolerate exceptions. We shall never ask for permission for doing the right thing.

This simple dogmatic approach is 100% under our own personal control. It's not mandated or supervised by regulatory compliance protocols. And, yeah, it doesn't come in an easy-to-digest pill.

It's a pure (un)common sense ethical obligation. One that is easy to learn, easy to practice, easy to role model, easy to teach, easy to monitor, easy to correct and mend, and easy to sustain over an entire surgical career.

Let me give you a few specific examples to make my point.

As the head of our department I sometimes have to consider myself the 'fixer' or 'psychoanalyst' for a multiplicity of ad-hoc issues, unprecedented problems and individual complaints that originate on a daily basis at our busy high-volume and high-acuity level 1 trauma center (that is, unless I 'hide' in green scrubs in the OR — unequivocally a surgeon's favorite escape from the daily hassles, meetings, and other annoyances).

A few years ago, a colleague of mine who specializes in reattaching traumatically amputated limbs, hands, and fingers (so-called "microvascular replantation surgery") stormed into my office, visibly upset, face flushed with anger.

My colleague stuttered with a trembling voice:

"Boss, this is horrendous, outrageous, and absolutely unacceptable!"

My standard screening phrase came into play:

"What happened? How can I help you?"

"Well, 2 hours ago I got a phone call from the ED about a young patient with a crushed thumb needing immediate surgery. Two hours! And the patient is still not in the OR!"

I understood that time was of the essence. Our protocol mandates that these patients must be streamlined to the OR as an acute "limb salvage" emergency, without any delay.

"Wow, that's crazy!" I said, "Let's run down to the OR bridge to figure out where the holdup is!" (For non-surgeons; the OR bridge is the generic designation for the 'command center' of the operating rooms.)

"No, no, you don't get it, that's not the problem!" my colleague clarified. "The problem is that our intern dropped the ball!"

"What happened?"

"I called the intern immediately after I got the alert and asked him to speed up getting the patient to the OR – but this didn't happen! The intern is still walking around with the add-on sheet, 2 hours after my phone call."

"Okay, okay," I said, "Let me figure this out and fix it for you right away!"

As I walked down to the OR bridge, I bumped into our intern who was running up from the ED, out of breath, carrying three different pagers and a stack of papers including dozens of H&Ps from additional consults. Plus, between all these papers was the ominous add-on sheet for the replantation case.

He apologized profusely and accepted full responsibility (as all interns do by default) for the delay in adding the case on. I just couldn't find a way to blame him. How should an intern be able to multi-task and prioritize all the assignments in light of the multiplicity of simultaneous urgent consults and requests?

I checked with the OR charge nurse and she gave us an immediate "go". The OR team was on stand-by and ready to take the patient to our dedicated urgent room. It took about 2 minutes for me to accomplish the task. All that was required was a short in-person, face-to-face discussion with the team. Done.

I checked back with my colleague: "Did you personally ensure with the charge nurse to get an immediate room? Sounds like the patient could have rolled back 2 hours ago? Is this a microvascular emergency or just a simple debridement?"

"I don't know," my colleague said, "I haven't seen the patient yet..."

"What?!"

"I went home for lunch and was walking my dog when I got the call. Seriously, I can't believe interns are so unreliable these days!"

Wow!

I was speechless.

What happened to Churchill's call to "never surrender"?

Where are the noble knights of the 21st century?

The ancient Greek philosopher and scientist Aristotle (384-322 BC) coined a classic quote on personal accountability: "We are what we repeatedly do. Excellence, then, is not an art, but a habit."

Hopefully, opting out of personally seeing a patient is not a new habit characteristic of the modern-age surgeon.

In closure of this anecdotal story, you will clearly understand that I was extremely empathetic (or rather, sympathetic) towards the intern in this situation. As I attested in the first chapter of the book, I've personally 'been there'. Interns take an oath to go through hell for a full year and to accept blame for anything that goes wrong, independent of whether they have been physically present or involved at all. In my 20+ years of surgical training and practice, I have personally witnessed the recent paradigm shift from a culture of 'blame & shame' to system safety.

We have now adopted a new pseudo-culture where 'The System' is supposed to keep our patients safe.

Well, guess what?

It's just not happening.

In my view, the pendulum has swung too far. The overwhelming load of regulatory compliance regulations, rules and protocols allows us to comfortably hide behind 'The System' (see Part 4 of the book). We are now in the luxurious position to grade any complication that leads to patient harm as a system failure.

This is, of course, the natural short-cut. We've transitioned from the dark ages when surgeons used to work more than 100 hours per week to a new modern age where working past 5pm to serve our patients is considered a gallant and nearly heroic act. Really, it's gotten ridiculous. ("Last night I saw my partner Mark Hammerberg rounding on his total joint patients at 8pm. He must be nuts!")

Let's put this alleged 'immense workload' for surgeons into a bit of perspective. Pardon me. I just have to go there.

Census data from 2012 show the median annual wage in the United States at $26,695 per person, with two-thirds of all Americans earning less than $40,000 per year. In sharp contrast, the 2012 average U.S. physician salaries published by *Forbes Magazine* revealed that even the lowest-paid doctors (family practitioners, pediatricians, and psychiatrists) earn an average base pay of $189,000 a year (seven times the median wage). These numbers appear pale compared to surgeons' average salaries. Not including productivity incentives, bonuses and benefits, a general surgeon makes $349,791 a year (13 times the median wage), $461,000 for urologists (17 times), $519,000 for orthopedic surgeons (19 times), and $760,782 for spine surgeons (28 times).

Granted, we go through a lengthy training and bear an immense responsibility both for our patients and for ourselves. For example, I've personally spent a total of 11 years in training after medical school, including internship, residency and fellowships. Still, when we compare ourselves to Siberian coal miners, we drastically overstate our own 'pseudo-suffering'.

To assure you I'm not making this stuff up for my own convenience, I'll pass on the word of a real coal miner 'in the trenches' (or better: 'in the tunnels').

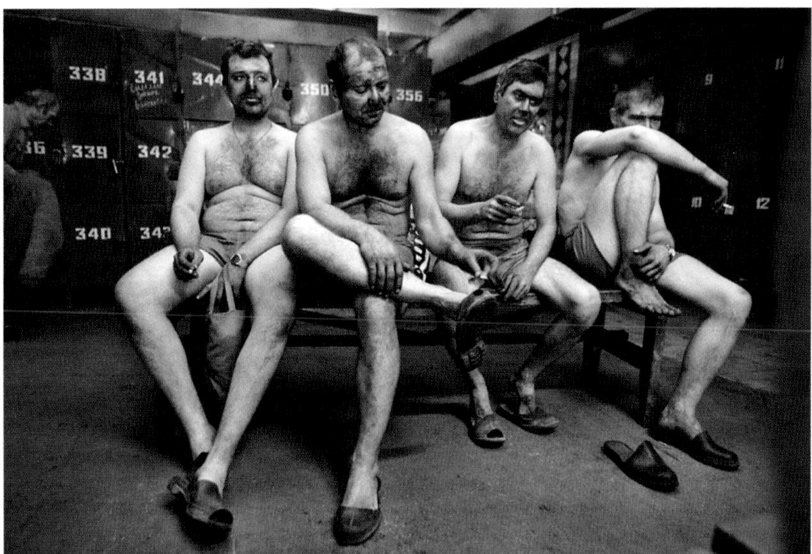

21st century Siberian coal miners, during a break from work. © Jacob Ehrbahn/POLFOTO/PA Images.

Anatoly Malikhin, a young tunneller from Novokuznetsk, a city of 550,000 in south-western Siberia, recently spoke up at the Russian Congress of People's Deputies to request better working conditions for coal miners (Table 3).

Table 3. A coal miner's story.

- "This is not a life for human beings. We have no time for leisure. We have no decent clothes. We spend our entire lives making just enough money to feed ourselves and our children. The day shift starts at 6am, so you have to be up at 4:30am. You go to the mine, work 8 hours underground, and all your life is work. When you come home you are too exhausted to do anything but collapse. On the weekend there are chores to do at home. About the only leisure we have is a mug or two of beer in the morning after a night shift. That's it. And then you quit — if you haven't already been killed in an accident. A few years later, your lungs give out, or your heart goes. Bye-bye. You're dead."

I know, I know. You're thinking this example is too exotic and far-fetched to be potentially relevant for us, right? Well, just look around in our own practice. For example, take a peek at my janitor friend, David Frein, who empties the trash in my office every day. First, you have to understand that a janitor's average salary in the United States in 2013 was $22,590 (i.e. $4,000 below the median annual wage). Then, you have to consider that David indeed works Siberian coal miner's hours.

You don't believe me? Well, I've asked him!

David works two full-time jobs in parallel. He has no choice. David has to feed his family, support his wife and two stepchildren, and take care of his bedridden mother who lives with them at their small two-bedroom condominium near our hospital in Denver. His mother requires 24/7 nursing support and, obviously, David cannot afford to pay for an expensive qualified care facility. In all his modesty, David would never complain about his quality of life or work. Actually, it took me several years of bonding and building a personal relationship until I dared to inquire about his specific work schedule and to understand how David is able to make ends meet.

Here, in a nutshell, is David's daily life: he gets up at 5am every day to start his work at Denver Health by 6am (roughly the same shift as a Siberian coal miner). After a full day of work cleaning floors and hallways and emptying hundreds of trashcans (including the one in my office), he finishes his day job around 2pm and drives to a Denver public school. There he starts his second job, cleaning the school from 4pm until midnight. David admits to occasionally taking a short 30-minute nap in his car, pulling off to the side of the road during the commute between the two jobs. When he gets home well after midnight, he takes a shower, eats his main meal of the day, and climbs into bed beside his sleeping wife.

As David tells me: "You know, doctor, I typically can't sleep right away after working non-stop for 18 hours, so I just relax and take some time to read and think..."

Often, he picks up a Saturday or Sunday shift to be able to pay his bills.

Incredible perseverance, right?

I have so much respect for the hard workers in our community. I lack any suitable words.

Oh, by the way, my other janitor friend, Mike McClain (the man who cleans our operating rooms), recently told me that he works *three* full-time jobs. I didn't even know that was humanly possible!

So do we still consider it 'crazy' for surgeons to occasionally round on our patients after 8pm? Or is it perhaps crazy that we feel entitled to walk our dog at home during a 2-hour lunch break?

Of note, my janitor friend David Frein doesn't walk his dog for two reasons:

(1) He can't afford to own one; and (2) He never takes a lunch break.

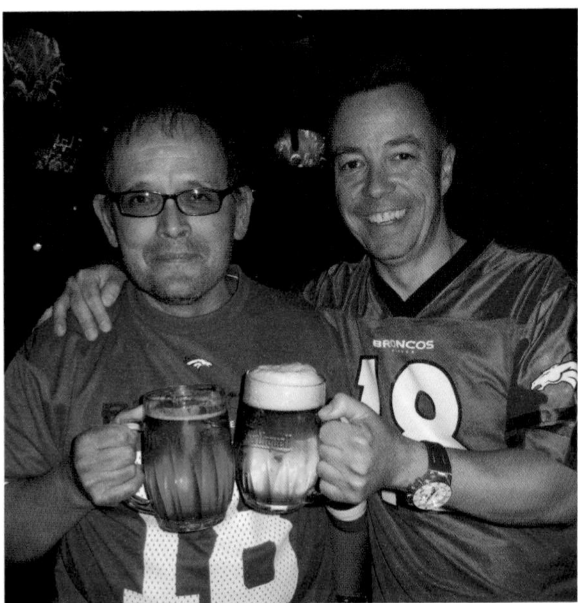

With my janitor friend David Frein on a rare occasion when he was off work on a Sunday. I took the opportunity to invite David for beers to watch the Denver Broncos defeat the Green Bay Packers on November 1, 2015.

Let me finalize this discussion by offering an example of a pragmatic approach to measuring the extent of surgeons' individual accountability: hand hygiene compliance.

Isn't this a perfect surrogate marker of "doing the right thing" for our patients at all times?

I recently challenged a young and enthusiastic third-year medical student who rotated through our outpatient clinic. We discussed a case in detail and, before walking back to see the patient, I asked him:

"Are you ready to save some lives today?"

He answered without hesitation: "Yessir, absolutely!"

"What I meant to ask is whether *you* are going to save some lives today?"

I got a blank stare. "With all due respect, sir, I can't save any lives; I am just a medical student!"

"*Just* a medical student?" I replied, "You're an adult human being willing to dedicate the rest of your life to your patients and your community as a healer and servant. That's exactly what you are and nothing less. So I'm asking you one more time: Are *you* going to save some lives today?"

"I am not sure... How can I do that, sir?"

I urged him to follow me down the hall to see our patient. Before we entered the room, I stopped both of us in front of the examination room and pointed to the antiseptic foam dispenser.

"This is how you can save dozens or hundreds of lives every day, starting today, for the rest of your career!" I said as I smiled and took two clicks of the sanitizing foam and rubbed the palm of my hands. "Did you know that there are nearly one million preventable, hospital-acquired infections in U.S. hospitals every year? And that we kill about 75,000 to 100,000 of these patients annually with our self-created infections?"

My med student continued his bemused stare, so I pursued the educational module: "Can you believe that around one in every 25 patients seeking medical treatment at a hospital acquires a new infection? These include infections of the lungs and bowels, bloodstream infections after central venous line placement, and catheter-associated urinary tract infections. And guess what? As surgeons, in the United States, we create around 160,000 postoperative surgical site infections every year!"

"I wasn't aware of that. I clearly didn't go into medicine to harm any patients..."

"Right on, that's exactly my point! Have you ever heard of *C. diff.*?"

"No, sir."

"*C. diff.* stands for *Clostridium difficile*, which earned its Latin adjective due to its property of being extremely difficult to eradicate. This bacterium causes so-called 'pseudomembranous colitis', a severe infection of the colon that originates as a side effect of antibiotics that we give to our patients every day. *C. diff.* alone is responsible for about 30,000 in-hospital deaths every year. And guess how it's transmitted from one person to the other?"

"Through the fecal-oral route?"

"Indeed. That's why we have an easy way to deal with this 'difficult' pathogen: to wash our hands! Every time you opt out, you deliberately permit the chance that one of your patients may die from a preventable infection. Therefore: never make an exception!"

"Wow. Thank you, sir. I never thought about it from that perspective."

Somewhat proud of my compelling argument and feeling I'd just converted another medical student to the right cause, I took an additional two clicks of hand sanitizing foam, ensured that my young colleague did the same, knocked on the exam room door and entered the patient's room.

I actually confront every medical student assigned to my supervision with this simple mind game. And guess what? The students get it.

Yet, despite the incontrovertible impact of hand hygiene as a simple core measure that could potentially save tens of thousands of patients' lives every year, surgeons generally don't tend to take this precaution very seriously. It's a hassle. It's an afterthought. Plus, surgeons generally don't appreciate administrators telling them what to do.

Believe it or not, there are researchers who study hand hygiene rates in hospitals and clinics. These rates are generally calculated as the ratio of the performed action (hand sanitizer usage) to the number of opportunities available (before entering and after exiting a patient room).

Published estimates show that the overall hand hygiene compliance in health care across the globe is around 30%.

You read that right. *Thirty percent.*

Despite being extremely proud of my own institution as one of the premier safety net hospitals in the country, and a forefront role model for embracing an open culture of patient safety, I am ashamed to admit that our own hand hygiene compliance is barely any better than the global average.

Guess how high our hand hygiene rate is at Denver Health when we feel as though no one's watching us?

Less than 40%!

This is even lower than the published average hand hygiene compliance rates at medical centers in Vietnam (47%),[22] Egypt (53%),[23] or Nigeria (65%).[24]

---

22 Salmon S, *et al.* Beginning the journey of hand hygiene compliance monitoring at a 2,100-bed tertiary hospital in Vietnam. *American Journal of Infection Control* 2014; 42: 71-3.

23 Amazian K, *et al.* Multicentre study on hand hygiene facilities and practice in the Mediterranean area: results from the NosoMed Network. *The Journal of Hospital Infection* 2006; 62: 311-8.

24 Uneke CJ, *et al.* Promotion of hand hygiene strengthening initiative in a Nigerian teaching hospital: implication for improved patient safety in low-income health facilities. *Brazilian Journal of Infectious Diseases* 2014; 18: 21-7.

Ironically, the compliance rates at Denver Health increase dramatically to more than 90% when we are officially observed and monitored.

This phenomenon likely relates to what has been dubbed the "Hawthorne effect". This basically outlines how a subject's behavior changes as a result of being observed. And the concept reflects very poorly on our individual accountability as surgeons!

The Hawthorne effect (also termed "observer effect" or "observation bias") derives its designation from studies performed in the 1920s and 1930s at the Hawthorne factory of the Western Electric Company in Illinois.

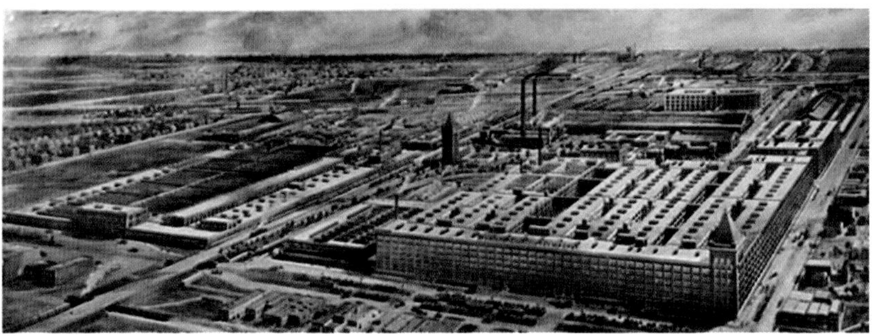

The Hawthorne Works, Cicero, IL (1925).

These early studies were designed to investigate the plant workers' productivity with varying light intensity inside the factory. When observed by researchers, workers' productivity dramatically increased and fell back to baseline levels when the study ended and the observers left.

Sounds like a no-brainer now, but it was the first time this phenomenon had been recognized. The studies also showed that workers increased their productivity independent of the changes that were implemented at the factory, as long as they felt they were being observed. A recent paper from the medical literature investigated the impact of the Hawthorne effect on hand hygiene compliance at an academic medical center in Toronto,

Ontario, Canada.[25] The set-up of the investigation was based on a location-tracking system that allowed for measuring hand hygiene product usage in real time. This extravagant system continuously monitors the location of health care workers, using a network of wireless receivers in patient rooms and hallways, as well as on hand sanitizer dispenser units across the inpatient ward (see the figure below from the original publication). The study results showed a dramatic increase in dispenser usage (three-fold) when official auditors were in close proximity, as compared to control observations in the absence of visible auditors. Ironically, this effect was not observed inside patient rooms where no auditors were present at any time.

Ah, we go back full circle to 'The System'.

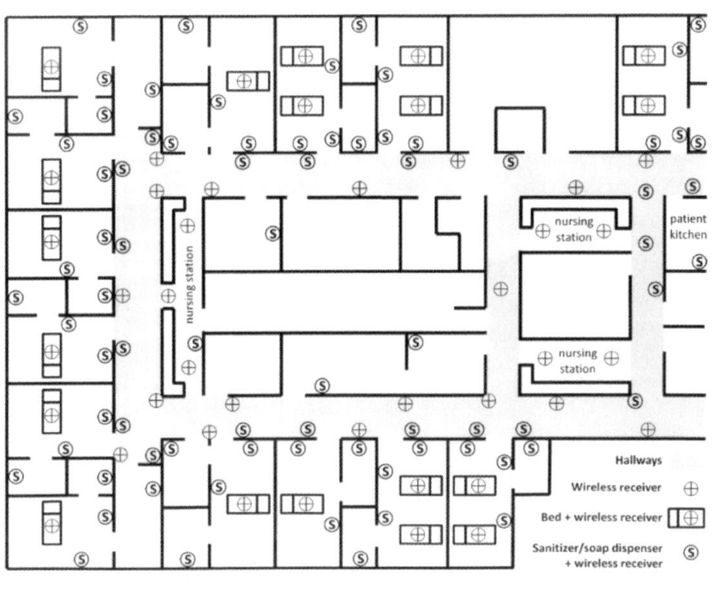

Unit floor plan and location of real-time location system components. Reprinted with permission from: Srigley JA, *et al. BMJ Qual Saf* 2014; 23: 974-80. (Creative Commons Attribution License, BMJ Publishing Group, Ltd.)

[25] Srigley JA, *et al.* Quantification of the Hawthorne effect in hand hygiene compliance monitoring using an electronic monitoring system: a retrospective cohort study. *BMJ Quality & Safety* 2014; 23: 974-80.

Perhaps a perfect system can provide staff training programs and logistic support, including door signs, checklists, and hand sanitizer dispensers inside and outside of patient rooms and across hallways on each ward. But in the absence of physician-driven individual accountability, the expected goal of 100% hand hygiene compliance remains utopian.

How is it possible that low-wage workers in the meat packing industry are able to sustain 100% compliance with hand hygiene protocols? It should be noted that a meat packers' salary is below the median wage ($24,190 in 2011) and in a similar range as my janitor friend David Frein's annual income. How are these poorly remunerated hard workers so extremely committed to "doing the right thing" – as opposed to us surgeons?

Of note, the meat-packing industry in the United States employs more than 100,000 workers and is considered to be one of the most hazardous industries in the country, both for workers and for consumers. Yet, they all wash their hands religiously.

When you buy fresh meat at the grocery store, you don't want to play Russian roulette. You want to rest assured with 100% confidence that the meat is not contaminated with *E. coli*, *Salmonella* or *Listeria*.

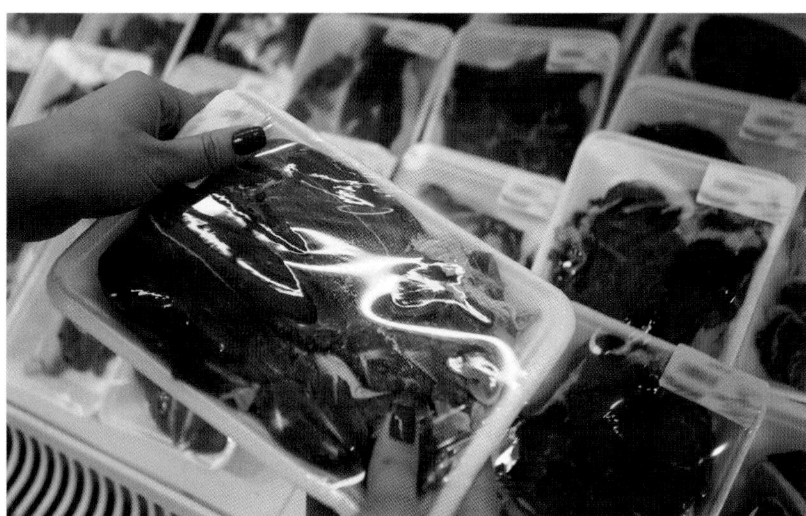

Strikingly, consumer confidence in meat safety is remarkably high, similar to our level of confidence when boarding a commercial plane. The regulatory compliance protocols by the Department of Agriculture's Food Safety Inspection Service (see Table 4)[26] are impressive and more restrictive than current CDC guidelines or Joint Commission protocols that regulate health workers' hand hygiene.

Table 4. **Hand hygiene requirements for meat packers.**[26]

- **416.5 Employee Hygiene:**
  - (a) Cleanliness. All persons working in contact with product, food-contact surfaces, and product-packaging materials must adhere to hygienic practices while on duty to prevent adulteration of product.
  - (b) Clothing. Aprons, frocks, and other outer clothing worn by persons who handle product must be of material that is disposable or readily cleaned. Clean garments must be worn at the start of each working day and garments must be changed during the day as often as necessary to prevent contamination or adulteration of product.
  - (c) Disease control. Any person who has or appears to have an infectious disease, open lesion, including boils, sores, or infected wounds, or any other abnormal source of microbial contamination must be excluded from any operations which could result in product adulteration until the condition is corrected.

- **2-301.11 Clean Condition:**
  Food employees shall keep their hand and exposed portions of their arms clean.

- **2-301.12 Cleaning Procedure:**
  - (a) Except as specified in (b) of this section, food employees shall clean their hands and exposed portions of their arms with a cleaning compound in a lavatory that is equipped as specified under 5-202.12 by vigorously rubbing together the surfaces of their lathered hands and arms for at least 20 seconds and thoroughly rinsing with clean water. Employees shall pay particular attention to the areas underneath the fingernails and between the fingers.

Continued overleaf

[26] www.fsis.usda.gov/OPPDE/rdad/FRPubs/San_Guide.pdf.

Table 4. Hand hygiene requirements for meat packers.[26]

(b) If approved and capable of removing the types of soils encountered in the food operations involved, an automatic handwashing facility may be used by food employees to clean their hands.

- **2-301.14 When to Wash:**
  Food employees shall clean their hands and exposed portions of their arms as specified under 2-301.12 immediately before engaging in food preparation including working with exposed food, clean equipment and utensils, and unwrapped single-service and single-use articles and:
  (a) After touching bare human body parts other than clean hands and clean, exposed portions of arms;
  (b) After using the toilet room;
  (c) After caring for or handling service animals or aquatic animals;
  (d) After coughing, sneezing, using a handkerchief or disposable tissue, using tobacco, eating, or drinking;
  (e) After handling soiled equipment or utensils;
  (f) During food preparation, as often as necessary to remove soil and contamination and to prevent cross contamination when changing tasks;
  (g) When switching between working with raw food and working with ready-to-eat food;
  (h) After engaging in other activities that contaminate the hands.

- **2-301.15 Where to Wash:**
  Food employees shall clean their hands in a handwashing lavatory or approved automatic handwashing facility and may not clean their hands in a sink used for food preparation, or in a service sink or a curbed cleaning facility used for the disposal of mop water and similar liquid waste.

- **2-301.16 Hand Sanitizers:**
  A hand sanitizer and a chemical hand sanitizing solution used as a hand dip shall comply with one of the following:
  (a) Be an approved drug that is listed in the FDA publication Approved Drug Products with Therapeutic Equivalence Evaluations as an approved drug based on safety and effectiveness; or

Continued overleaf

Table 4. Hand hygiene requirements for meat packers.[26]

(b) Have active antimicrobial ingredients that are listed in the FDA monograph for OTC Health-Care Antiseptic Drug Products as an antiseptic handwash; or

(c) Have components that are exempted from the requirement of being listed in federal food additive regulations as specified in 21 CFR 170.39 — Threshold of regulation for substances used in food-contact articles; or

(d) Comply with and be listed in:
- 21 CFR 178 — Indirect Food Additives: Adjuvants, Production Aids, and Sanitizers as regulated for use as a food additive with conditions of safe use, or
- 21 CFR 182 — Substances Generally Recognized as Safe, 21 CFR 184 — Direct Food Substances Affirmed as Generally Recognized as Safe, or 21 CFR 186 — Indirect Food Substances Affirmed as Generally Recognized as Safe for use in contact with food; and
- Be applied only to hands that are cleaned as specified under 2-301.12.

If a hand sanitizer or a chemical hand sanitizing solution used as a hand dip does not meet the criteria specified in this section, use shall be:

(a) Followed by thorough hand rinsing in clean water beforehand contact with food or by the use of gloves; or

(b) Limited to situations that involve no direct contact with food by the bare hands.

(c) A chemical hand sanitizing solution used as a hand dip shall be maintained clean and at a strength equivalent to at least 100mg/L chlorine.

- **2-302.11 Fingernail Maintenance:**

(a) Food employees shall keep their fingernails trimmed, filed and maintained so the edges and surfaces are cleanable and not rough.

(b) Unless wearing intact gloves in good repair, a food employee may not wear fingernail polish or artificial fingernails when working with exposed food.

- **2-303.11 Jewelry Prohibition:**

While preparing food, food employees may not wear jewelry on their arms and hands. This section does not apply to a plain ring such as a wedding band.

Philosophically, I feel like I'm somewhat of a meat packer. Yet I don't need those sophisticated guidelines for my own hand hygiene. My solution is simple. For many years, I've played a successful game, of which the odds are always in my favor: I offer our house staff and medical students who round with me on patient wards a $20 bill every time they catch me not using the hand sanitizer dispenser before entering and after exiting a patient room.

I've never had to pay once.

I never will.

Why?

Because I make no exceptions.

And I never ask for permission for doing the right thing.

PART 3
The safe patient

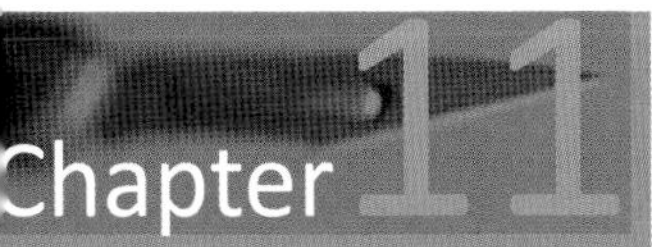

Chapter 11 The "eat-what-you-kill" phenomenon: how to avoid avoidable care

"It's hard to get a man to understand something when his salary depends upon his not understanding it!"

Upton Sinclair, Jr. (1878-1968)

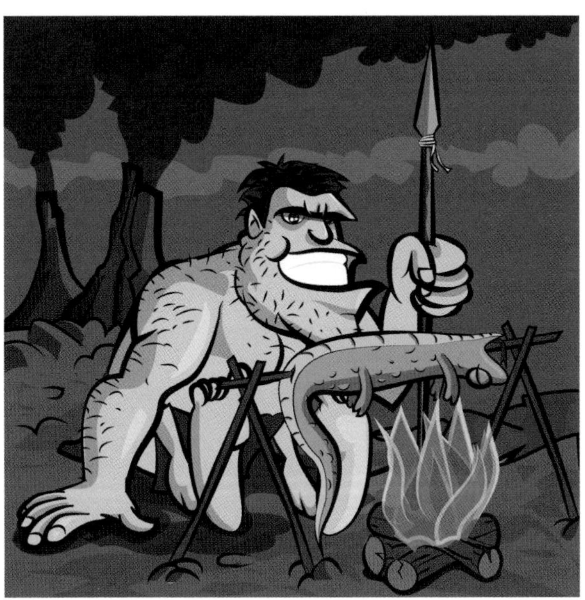

At some point in your life, no matter how healthy you are and how 'risk-free' you live, you're going to be admitted to the hospital. It's just a fact of modern life.

The truth is: human bodies are intrinsically vulnerable. We suffer from acute or chronic diseases, we're injured in accidents, and ultimately — with 100% probability over a lifetime and all odds against us — we die.

In fact, as a trauma surgeon, I witness, first-hand, how fast and unexpectedly bad things can happen. Most of the injuries I see in our ED require immediate hospitalization and urgent or emergent surgery; many have the potential for life-long impairment or death.

Pragmatically speaking, most of us will eventually step through the giant glass doors of a hospital, not as a visitor or health care provider, but as a patient. And the uncontested expectation when one enters a hospital is to be better off after being discharged than at the time of admission.

In the absence of this incentive, most people would never set foot in a hospital voluntarily. Or would you?

But what if it was worse? What if patients knew *a priori* that they wouldn't do any better after surgical treatment? Or if they were told that they'd suffer additional harm, experience complications, or contract new diseases; that they would leave the hospital in a wheelchair or in a coffin?

Yikes!

How many people would step through those glass doors then?

Think about your expectations when you step onto a commercial aircraft. You clearly don't expect to crash and die, otherwise you'd go for a different transportation option. Train, anyone? How about when you order a *Nigiri* dish at your favorite sushi place? You don't place your order expecting to contract a parasite or another preventable infection. You don't consider eating sushi to be a game of Russian roulette. If you did, you'd rather have dinner at the Italian place around the corner.

Your justified expectation is to be 100% safe when boarding a commercial plane or when ordering raw seafood at the sushi bar. How safe are you supposed to feel when entering the hospital door as a patient?

Most people consider hospitals safe. Incredibly safe.

The general population would never expect that anything bad could happen to them in a hospital. After all, health care staff are exclusively trained to use their healing hands and extensive knowledge to restore people's health. In most minds, a hospital is a building where you go in sick and walk out healed.

Sadly, this idea is an illusion.

In the United States alone more than a million people admitted to a hospital will develop a new infection while staying there, and up to 100,000 of them will die from that newly acquired disease every year.[27] That's a staggering number.

To put this into perspective, the annual rate of preventable deaths during hospitalization in the United States is more than 30-fold the number of innocent victims killed in the terrorist attacks of September 11, 2001.

And those stats are repeated every year!

There is no Patriot Act legislation on the horizon designed to protect our patients from unnecessary harm. No cavalry to the rescue.

So what can patients do to protect themselves from the hidden dangers of our health care system? The most pragmatic approach to avoid complications originating from medical treatment is to question whether the treatment is required at all.

27 www.cdc.gov/HAI/surveillance/.

Maybe we need another dictum: to strictly avoid avoidable care.

Hang on, what do I mean by "avoidable care"?

In surgery, I define this as any surgical intervention that was either not needed in the first place, or was not in the patient's best interest when balanced against other available treatment options. In other words: I'm talking about "unneeded surgery".

You think it doesn't happen?

Unfortunately, this is more frequent than patients (and surgeons) appreciate.

Let's spend a minute looking at an example from my own experience.

When I trained as a resident in orthopaedic trauma surgery in Europe, I was taught many dogmatic surgical tenets. One example of an unquestioned surgical indication included the notion that so-called "syndesmotic screws" for fixation of unstable ankle fractures must be removed in a second surgery in all cases.

No questions asked.

For years, we took 100% of these patients back to the operating room within 6 to 12 weeks after the first surgery for a "mandatory" removal of those ankle transfixation screws. As a dedicated resident in training, I hardly questioned the doctrine. In contrast, I was one of the hospital's minions who enthusiastically explained to my patients why they strictly needed a subsequent surgical procedure.

It was only after I moved to the United States years later that I realized how many of our dogmatic surgical indications were unfounded. In Denver, none of my partners were compelled to remove syndesmotic screws after ankle fracture fixation. And guess what? Their patients appeared to be doing very well without undergoing a second surgery.

Somewhat confused and unsettled, I asked my rotating German research fellow at the time, Sebastian Weckbach, to investigate this conundrum based on our extensive fracture database at Denver Health.

Sebastian spent several months searching for all patients with ankle fractures repaired by syndesmotic screw fixation during a 5-year time period. The result of his research was truly mind-boggling: in a total cohort of 140 consecutive patients, only two individuals (1.4%) had symptoms related to syndesmotic screws that required a subsequent surgical procedure for elective screw removal.

Two patients!

The remaining 138 patients did not have any symptoms related to the screws even in circumstances where follow-up radiographs showed signs of screw motion, screws bending, or even screws breaking.

Holy shit!

I felt horrible!

Our study showed that more than 98% of all patients did not require a second surgical procedure. Yet, during my entire surgical training in Europe, we removed syndesmotic screws in all patients.

Right, all of them. Every single one, without exception.

Talk about an example of systematic unnecessary surgery.

In retrospect, I felt like I had been an accomplice to a system-wide conspiracy bent on pushing our patients into unjustified surgery with no benefits. The first thing Sebastian and I did as an immediate action item was to publish our study in the German literature to spread the word.[28]

---

[28] Weckbach S, *et al.* Ist das routinemässige Belassen von Syndesmosenschrauben nach operativer Versorgung instabiler Sprunggelenksfrakturen gerechtfertigt? Erfahrung eines US-Traumazentrums an 140 konsekutiven Patienten. *Zeitschrift für Orthopädie und Unfallchirurgie* 2014; 152: 554-7.

It should be noted that at the time of my drafting this book chapter, the removal of syndesmotic screws was still recommended as a "standard of care" in the German AO Manual — the 'bible' for orthopaedic trauma care — and by guidelines from the German Academy for Medical Sciences (AWMF).[29]

While the general risks from undergoing a simple screw removal are minimal, occasional major complications have been described. These include the occurrence of a new fracture after syndesmotic screw removal [30] and a surprisingly high wound infection rate around 9% after the subsequent (unnecessary) procedure.[31]

I couldn't help but remember the case of a very nice elderly lady who developed an uncontrolled surgical site infection after we removed her syndesmotic screw. After multiple surgical revisions and weeks of unneeded suffering, she ended up losing her leg.

True story.

She had an amputation secondary to an unneeded surgery.

Maybe you're saying that I'm blowing this problem out of proportion simply based on a single poor-quality retrospective study performed by our own group? Fair enough. I actually use this argument all the time when debating over the published literature with my colleagues. I will put aside the syndesmotic screw riddle and instead challenge you with a real brain teaser. Let's focus on the most commonly performed surgical procedure in the world: arthroscopic partial meniscectomy.

This minimally-invasive surgical procedure allows a surgeon to examine and treat internal knee damage through two small 'buttonhole' incisions. The apparent advantage of the technique is that you don't have

---

29 AWMF Leitlinie Nr. 021/003, 2011 (www.awmf.org).

30 Citak M, *et al.* Distal tibia fracture post syndesmotic screw removal: an adverse complication. *Archives of Orthopaedic and Trauma Surgery* 2011; 131: 1405-8.

31 Schepers T, *et al.* Complications of syndesmotic screw removal. *Foot & Ankle International* 2001; 32: 1040-4.

to surgically expose the knee joint through a conventional open approach (arthrotomy).

In a nutshell, the purpose of performing an arthroscopic partial meniscectomy is to relieve acute or chronic symptoms attributed to a tear in the meniscus by removing torn fragments and trimming the meniscus into a more stable shape. The benefits of this outpatient procedure are intuitive. The postoperative recovery period is short (due to the small surgical stab incisions) and patients regain function very quickly.

However, this routine procedure is hardly routine if you consider the risk of a postoperative complication (actually, no surgical procedure should ever be termed "routine" — it's quite the opposite from the patient's perspective!).

Let's brain-storm about the 'bad stuff' that could happen to a patient after a simple knee scope: a severe infection of the knee (septic arthritis); a blood clot to the veins of the leg (DVT) with potential migration of the clot into the lungs (PE); and the latter, of course, bears the risk of a potentially fatal outcome — from the hospital directly to the morgue, after a routine outpatient procedure.

Now here's the wake-up call: in the United States alone approximately 700,000 patients have an arthroscopic partial meniscectomy performed every year. Even with a low conservative estimate of an overall complication rate of 1% to 2% (the 'standard' risk prediction), around 7,000 to 14,000 patients will suffer a complication. And a few extremely unfortunate patients may actually *die* from a fatal PE.

Now dig this: what if I told you that an arthroscopic partial meniscectomy has no proven benefits at all? Your spontaneous reaction might be to question my mental sanity. I don't hold it against you. Just give me the time to challenge you with the results from a study published a couple of years ago.[32] The authors from the FIDELITY trial (Finnish Degenerative Meniscal Lesion Study) performed a prospective

[32] Sihvonen R, *et al.* Arthroscopic partial meniscectomy versus sham surgery for a degenerative meniscal tear. *New England Journal of Medicine* 2013; 369: 2515-24.

randomized double-blind controlled trial designed to evaluate the benefit of standard arthroscopic meniscal trimming versus sham surgery.

A total of 146 patients of age 35 to 65 years were enrolled who had clinical symptoms of a degenerative medial meniscus tear unresponsive to conventional treatment for at least 3 months (in the absence of a history of trauma or underlying osteoarthritis). Patients were randomly assigned to either arthroscopic partial meniscectomy or sham surgery. Random allocation was done by opening a concealed envelope in the operating room immediately prior to surgery. Patients were unaware of whether they had a partial meniscectomy performed or just a sham surgery.

Wanna take a shot at the results?

At 12 months' follow-up, there was *no difference* in outcome scores and extent of long-term knee pain between the two groups.

Seriously!

Let me say this in other words: those patients whose degenerative meniscus was left untreated had the same quality of subjective outcomes 1 year after surgery as those patients who underwent the meniscal trimming.

What I'm basically telling you is that one of the most frequently performed surgical procedures on the planet provides only risks and no benefits!

Do I have your full attention now?

But wait — there's more!

When I was a first-year intern in 1994, open appendectomy celebrated its centennial since the first description by Charles McBurney in 1894. This was the most frequent surgical 'training procedure' for residents, and we were all excited to sign up such cases during our call shifts. The technique of opening the abdominal wall to remove an inflamed appendix was considered the gold standard in the treatment of acute appendicitis.

For the next two decades, I followed the heated debate between advocates of 'New Age' minimally-invasive laparoscopic techniques and the conservative representatives of the traditional (open) McBurney procedure. This was a hot topic for keynote lectures and debate fora at surgical society meetings across the globe. I assume you have a premonition of where I'm going with this? The most recent debate is no longer dedicated to nuances in the surgical technique for removing inflamed appendices, but rather to the question of whether patients with uncomplicated appendicitis should be operated on at all.

In 2015, a landmark article from the multicenter randomized APPAC trial in Finland[33] revealed that 186 of 256 patients treated exclusively by antibiotics for CT-confirmed acute appendicitis did not require a surgical appendectomy during a 1-year follow-up period. In other words, 72.7% of all patients with uncomplicated appendicitis in the antibiotic treatment arm of the study were successfully cured without surgery.

Are you still with me?

You may look up any medical textbook of your choice for the treatment of acute appendicitis — it's an unequivocal surgical entity.

No uncertainty. Always operate.

Now consider that the antibiotic classes used in the APPAC trial[33] have been available on the market since the 1960s and 1970s. I don't even want to conceive how many millions of patients around the world have undergone unneeded appendectomies in the past decades.

Granted that we still have to understand the outcome of the selected 27.3% patients in the study who underwent a delayed appendectomy. These patents likely had an increased surgical complication rate due to local scar formation, chronic inflammation, and a risk of peritonitis from a delayed appendix perforation. Nevertheless, these recent data are clearly thought-provoking.

---

[33] Salminen P, *et al.* Antibiotic therapy vs. appendectomy for treatment of uncomplicated acute appendicitis: The APPAC randomized clinical trial. *JAMA* 2015; 313: 2340-8.

To finalize the discussion on avoidable surgery, let me shock you with a horrific example. There is a spine surgeon who recently made the news after being convicted for deliberately performing unnecessary spinal fusions as a 'standard practice' for pure financial gain (Table 5).

Table 5. News story reported by the Detroit Free Press (May 22, 2015): Birmingham doc admits to $11 million fraud for unneeded surgery.

- Neurosurgeon A.S. admitted performing unneeded spine operations. A Birmingham neurosurgeon pleaded guilty today to performing unnecessary spinal surgeries on patients and unlawfully billing the government and private insurance companies $11 million for the operations, the U.S. Attorney's office announced today. Dr. A.S. (39) entered guilty pleas in two separate cases before the U.S. Distric Judge (...), admitting he convinced patients to undergo spinal fusion surgeries with medical stabilizing devices that he actually never used, but billed public and private health care programs for it. (...) Dr. S. will be sentenced in September. Under the terms of his plea agreement, he faces between 9 and 11 years in prison. "This case of health care fraud is particularly egregious because Dr. S. caused serious bodily injury to his patients by acting out of his own greed instead of the best interest of his patients." U.S. Attorney (...) said in a statement. "Not only did he steal $11 million in insurance proceeds, but he also betrayed his trust to patients by lying to them about the procedures that were medically necessary and that were actually performed."

How can patients ever know when surgical indications are driven by a surgeon's own best interest — greed?

Let's leave this individual rogue surgeon in his prison cell (where he belongs) under the assumption that such unethical and criminal behavior only happens once in a million years.[34]

[34] Klaidman S. *Coronary - A True Story of Medicine Gone Awry*. New York, USA: Scribner, 2007.

Instead we will spend a minute on the question of "why". How on Earth is it possible that an ethical and reasonable surgeon would unconsciously perform unneeded surgeries? If I analyze the question pragmatically, I find two distinct reasons, which may actually feed into each other:

- *Reason 1*. We do surgery for a specific condition because that's what we've been trained to do; it's the way we've always done it, and we just don't know any better.
- *Reason 2*. We are incentivized to perform more surgical procedures, either for financial gain, renown, or both.

Regarding reason number 1:

This concept is called *Funktionslust*. The word is derived from German psychology and implies that living creatures like to do what they do best; dogs like to run, birds like to fly, dolphins like to swim, surgeons like to operate. It's intrinsic.

In positive psychology, this notion is reflected by "flow" which represents a state in which our level of skill and level of challenge completely match. This allows us to tap into a mental state driven by energized focus, full engagement, and enjoyment of the process of activity (i.e. surgery). In essence, "flow" describes a mental state of complete absorption in what we do.

Here's a personal example:

I fix around three to four ankle fractures every week. Those are the most common injuries seen in our emergency department. If you look at the schematic figure overleaf, you could argue that my own mismatch of skill level (high) versus challenge level (low) will put me in a state between *boredom* and *relaxation* whenever I fix a broken ankle. I'm sure you've been there too. None of my partners get too excited about fixing ankle fractures. Therefore, these routine injuries are typically relegated to more junior members of the team.

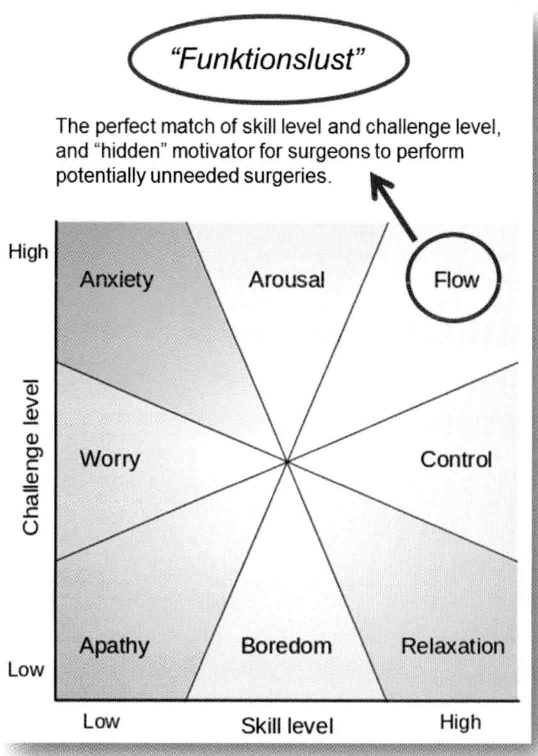

In contrast to ankle fractures, I absolutely enjoy fixing spine injuries and pelvic fractures. This is where my surgical skills and challenge match at the highest level (*flow*). The peak of my personal excitement is best represented by the clinical scenario where I can combine pelvic and spinal surgical techniques by connecting the pelvis to the lower lumbar spine with large-caliber screws and rods. This is called a "triangular osteosynthesis with lumbopelvic and iliosacral screw fixation".

Technically speaking, it's a lot of fun.

I bet that unconsciously my own inner *Funktionslust* drives me regularly to consider claiming such injuries presented at our morning conference. It's likely not a bad thing for a patient to be operated on by a surgeon who feels appropriately qualified to perform a specific procedure, as long as the indication is justified.

If you look at the figure above, you probably wouldn't want to go under the knife with a *bored* or *apathetic* surgeon, right?

Yet, having a triangular osteosynthesis of the pelvis performed is not always in the patient's best interest. The procedure is risky and associated with the potential for severe complications, including breakdown of the thin skin envelope over the back of the pelvis, misplacement of a pedicle screw into the spinal canal, and misplacement of the iliosacral screw into nerves and vessels. A highly skilled and experienced surgeon once told me of a case where a patient bled to death from an iliosacral screw placed into the superior gluteal artery. The patient subsequently died in the ICU due to delayed recognition of the exsanguinating internal hemorrhage (a close reminder of my first preventable patient death in 1994).

My personal trick to mitigate the unconsciously seductive power of *Funktionslust* is to be fully aware of this dangerous hidden motivator for surgery at all times.

Regarding reason number 2:

The second identified root cause of unnecessary surgery is probably more prevalent and harmful to our patients. This relates to surgeons' hidden (or apparent) incentives to perform surgical procedures, either for financial gain, renown, or both.

Our own ego drives us to perform as many particular procedures of interest as possible in order to increase professional respect among peers. The higher the caseload, the more we get to brag about it. Clearly, we want to be thought of as 'experts' in a specific field. This is best accomplished by impressing our competitors with a high volume and complexity of surgical cases. There's a pragmatic rule of thumb suggesting we should always divide the number of surgical cases — and multiply the number of complications — reported by a surgeon at least by a factor of three.

The 'expert reputation' incentive turns ominous when the volume of surgical procedures also provides a potential for financial gain. This is the clear and present danger for our patients today!

Let me elaborate: regardless of the type of practice (academic, hospital-based, or private office-based), most surgeons' salaries are driven by some kind of financial incentive linked to productivity, that is, the annual number and the 'size' of surgical cases.

For surgeons there are two main financial compensation models.

On the one hand, some surgeons are directly employed by hospitals on a flat annual salary. This is clearly the best-case scenario for any patient, as a surgeon's income remains steady independent of productivity and surgical volumes. The 'flat-salary surgeon' is therefore considered the safest surgeon from a patient's perspective, as there are no incentives to perform unnecessary surgeries. Unquestionably, a flat salary encourages a surgeon to exclusively provide appropriate care.

At Denver Health, for example, we are currently still employed as straight salaried surgeons. This means that neither my partners nor myself make a single cent more for performing a higher number of surgical procedures, seeing additional patients in clinic, or taking more 24/7 call shifts. This is likely the safest scenario for any patient under consideration for a surgical procedure. Under this routine, patients can therefore confidently assume that the recommended surgical care is of a real benefit for restoration of their health (instead of restoration of their surgeon's wallet).

Of note, the world-renowned Mayo Clinic in Rochester, Minnesota, follows the exact same model of flat-salaried physicians. Arguably, this may represent one of the underlying explanations of the Mayo Clinic's secret of success. Guaranteed patient outcomes based on flat-salary surgeons — sounds like a no-brainer!

On the other extreme side, there are surgeons in private practice models who are reimbursed almost exclusively for services provided. This is analogous to the 'commission only' model seen at a car dealership or furniture store. It's been provocatively termed the "eat-what-you-kill" phenomenon.

Imagine being beamed back to the Stone Age and think of private practice surgeons as hunting for survival. The model is quite simple: you get to bill for your services and keep the collections from patient encounters and surgical procedures. The harder you hunt, the more rewarding the bounty.

You don't think that's actually happening?

Well, let me challenge your good faith with a quote from Dr. Marty Makary's (must-read) bestseller, *Unaccountable*.[35] In the part of the book dedicated to financial incentives for surgeons, Marty provides the following egregious example:

> "Hospitals explicitly pressure their doctors to do more procedures and see more patients in order to make more money. One doctor I know received an email from his department that read: As we approach the end of the fiscal year, try to do more operations. Your productivity will be used to determine your bonus."

Do you think patients are aware of such financial incentives?

This is like being thrown into a health care market where you can't leave a surgeon's office without being scheduled for surgery, as much as you can't leave a car dealership without buying a new car.

Between the two basic reimbursement models (flat salary versus *eat-what-you-kill*) there is a common 'hybrid' model where physicians are salaried and have a certain component of their annual salary at risk, typically somewhere between 5% to 30%. The incentive remuneration is

[35] Makary M. *Unaccountable - What Hospitals Don't Tell You and How Transparency can Revolutionize Health Care*. New York, USA: Bloomsbury Press, 2012.

based on a certain amount of dollars paid per so-called "Relative Value Unit" (RVU), a standardized benchmark metric to determine the financial value of medical services provided and procedures performed.

Clearly, hospitals have a strong interest in having surgeons perform more procedures. In addition to the RVUs created by providers, hospitals get to bill for so-called "facility fees" for every surgical procedure. It comes as no surprise that hospital administrators spend millions of dollars to hire 'expert' consultants who tell us how to make more money by being more productive. This is a win-win both for hospitals and surgeons, as procedural billing codes are associated with higher RVUs than other physician activities, such as coordination of patient care, teaching residents, and performing research. Sadly, the important humanitarian aspects of our work as healers will quickly fall victim to the collateral damage inflicted by the demons of this business model.

So how can patients who enter a surgeon's office be confident that they really need a recommended surgical procedure? How can patients be assured that a proposed intervention truly represents the optimal treatment of choice? How can patients know that they won't be exposed to the learning curve of a new procedure or a young surgeon in training? How can they avoid exposure to the *Funktionslust* incentive of an expert senior surgeon? Or, worse, fall prey to the financial *eat-what-you-kill* incentive?

Bear with me, as we continue our journey towards understanding how better surgeons can build and sustain an infrangible partnership with their patients — and thereby make them safer.

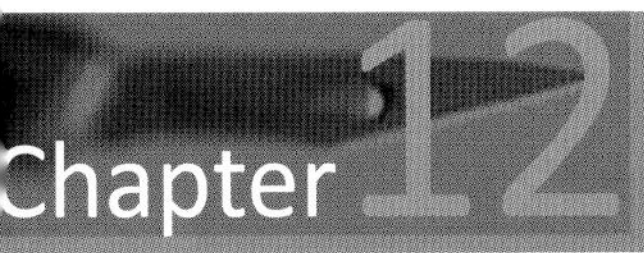

Chapter 12 Nothing about me, without me!

"I have an almost complete disregard of precedent, and a faith in the possibility of something better. It irritates me to be told how things have always been done. I defy the tyranny of precedent. I go for anything new that might improve the past."

Clara Barton (1821-1912)
Founder of the American Red Cross

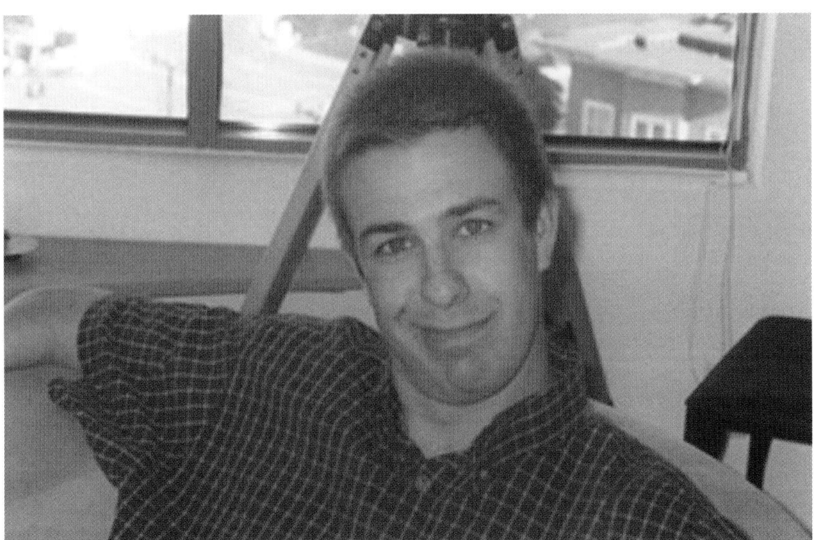

Michael Skolnik (March 15, 1979 — June 4, 2004). This is the last picture taken of Michael at age 22, before he underwent unnecessary brain surgery. There had been no pre-operative shared decision-making process or discussion of alternative treatment options. Michael died after nearly 3 years of agony and sequelae from multiple postoperative complications. (Photograph provided courtesy of Patty Skolnik.)

Imagine boarding a plane that you know will crash.

A horrible thought, right?

No one in his or her right mind would ever consider it.

And we won't really have to. Experts estimate the risk of dying in a plane crash is so extremely low that an individual could fly once a day consecutively for four million years before succumbing to a fatal crash. Now imagine the horrendous irony of dying in a plane crash after boarding the wrong flight. It's not too far-fetched if you substitute the airplane for a hospital. This scenario — mistakenly getting on a doomed flight — is comparable to a patient dying from a surgical procedure that was not needed in the first place.

I'll give you a true story.

The last normal day in Michael Skolnik's life began like any other. September 17th, 2001 was a hot summer day in Colorado. Michael was a 22-year-old EMT and nursing student spending the day at his parent's house. He was playing with their new puppy dog on the couch.

And then it happened.

Suddenly, unexpectedly.

Michael seized on the couch and passed out. He was rushed to the emergency room of a community hospital in the Denver Metro area. The ED docs initiated a standard diagnostic work-up by a CT scan and MRI. The findings in the radiology report revealed a "tiny round hyperdensity which may represent a very small colloid cyst, and does not appear to create any ventricular obstruction at this time".

The consulting neurosurgeon explained to Michael's parents, David and Patty Skolnik, that he had been lucky to survive the initial seizure. That being said, Michael needed surgery and it had to happen quickly.

The neurosurgeon left no room for uncertainty. "I need to operate in the next 48 hours or Michael will die." He comforted Michael and his parents by stating that the operation would be "very simple", basically a "walk in the park".

His exact words.

"I don't even need to go into the brain. All I'll do is excise the cyst."

The neurosurgical procedure was scheduled to take 3 hours. It took longer. Much longer. As the hours passed, Michael's parents desperately awaited news in the family waiting room. They paced. They silently wept. They held each other's hands and waited.

When the neurosurgeon finally walked in to the waiting room, 6½ hours later, he kneeled in front of Patty, pulled down his surgical cap, and said: "This is the worst year of my life."

Patty and David froze in panic and shock. David couldn't speak. Patty was barely able to stutter a question: "How is Michael?"

During the extensive surgical procedure, the neurosurgeon told them, he was unexpectedly unable to locate the colloid cyst. He claimed that he had to "manipulate" Michael's brain during the surgery in his attempts.

It was later revealed, during a court deposition, that the neurosurgeon had only performed one (1) such surgical procedure in his entire career.

Much later, after David and Patty had done their own extensive research, they learned that there had in fact been a much safer and minimally-invasive alternative treatment option available to treat Michael's condition. Specifically trained neurosurgeons are able to perform so-called "neuroendoscopic procedures" that allow the extraction of colloid cysts in the brain using high-resolution video cameras on thin endoscopes applied through small burrholes in the skull. This patient-friendly and safe treatment modality was then, and is still, offered as a standard procedure by many neurosurgical experts across the United States.

However, this appealing surgical option was never offered to Michael. Nor was it ever discussed with his family. Michael's parents had been completely unaware that half of his skull would be cracked open and removed during the "walk in the park" procedure.

There had been no shared decision-making process prior to surgery. Non-surgical options, such as close observation with repeat imaging of the brain to monitor the size of the colloid cyst, didn't enter the conversation. The only option offered to Michael was an urgent and apparently "life-saving" surgical procedure.

It gets worse: Michael was asked to sign the written informed consent form while he was alone and under the influence of powerful narcotics the night before the operation. His parents had just left for the night.

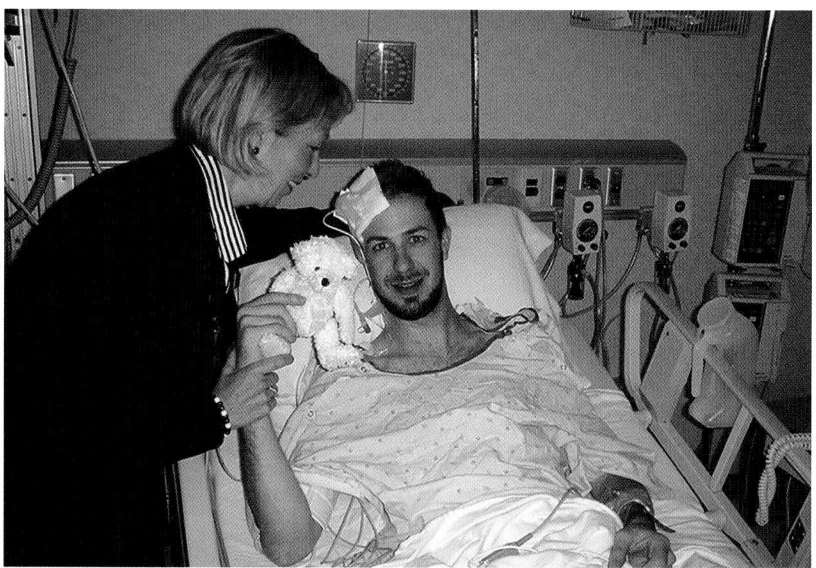

Michael Skolnik with his mother Patty at the bedside on the first night after his intraventricular drain had been placed. (Photograph provided courtesy of Patty Skolnik.)

The neurosurgeon's rush to surgery did not allow for sufficient time to even consider a second opinion (which was never offered anyway). It only became evident much later during court hearings that the neurosurgeon's pre-operative disclosure that he had done "multiple such routine procedures" turned out to be a simple and frank lie. The recommended operation had been entirely new to him.

The minor cyst extraction resulted in a cascade of life-threatening complications that landed Michael in an intensive care unit for 5 months. He developed a sequence of horrific adverse events including bleeding into the brain, recurring brain abscesses, hydrocephalus, pulmonary embolism, disseminated intravascular coagulation, hemiparalysis, psychosis, aphasia, partial blindness, thalamic chronic pain syndrome, recurring seizures, intracerebral yeast infection, MRSA infection, sepsis, multiple organ failure, and respiratory arrest.

Take a minute and read over that list again.

Think of this happening to one of your children. Or to any person among your loved ones. It's a pure nightmare. A horror show. And all of it is the result of a botched surgery.

None of the potential risks and complications had been discussed with Michael or his family prior to surgery.

No cyst was found or ever removed from Michael's brain.

The cold hard truth is, this young man had been exposed to an unnecessary brain surgery with 100% risk and 0% benefit.

After 32 months of endless suffering, on June 4, 2004, and confronted with yet another recurring complication, Michael gave up. He looked into his father's eyes, mouthed the words "I love you", and died.

In the decade following their son's preventable death, David and Patty Skolnik have traveled the globe as 'crusaders' for patient safety. Their mission is to dedicate the rest of their lives to ensuring that the voices of patients and their families are heard and taken seriously.

Shared decision-making for surgery should never be optional again.

Of note, Patty's tireless effort and lobbying for patient safety has led to the funding of the grassroots patient advocacy initiative "Citizens for Patient Safety" and to the passing of the Michael Skolnik Medical Transparency Act in Colorado.

In the United States alone, 22 million patients discuss the need for a surgical procedure with their surgeon every year. In addition, 75 million people make a decision about a new medication and around 100 million adults discuss the need for a diagnostic screening test during the same time frame.

To put this into a global perspective; about 200 million surgeries are performed worldwide every year. How many times do you think that patients and their families are truly involved in the surgical decision-making process? How many times are other treatment alternatives (including not having surgery) discussed in transparent detail? How many times are patients encouraged to seek a formal second opinion?

Let me challenge all surgeon readers with a 'moment of truth' question:

How likely are you to consider having a surgery done for yourself that you just recommended to one of your patients? In other words, do you treat your patients the same way you would treat yourself?

Do you think this question is too hypothetical to allow a coherent answer?

I don't think so!

The Science of Variation Group recently published a study designed to test this exact question.[36] The survey asked 254 participating surgeons to review a variety of clinical scenarios for which surgical treatment is optional, and to come up with a simple "yes/no" answer of whether they would recommend the surgery or not. The surgeons were furthermore asked to grade the confidence for their decision on a scale from 0 to 10 points. Half of the participants were randomly assigned to choose treatment for

[36] Janssen SJ, *et al.* Do surgeons treat their patients like they would treat themselves? *Clinical Orthopaedics and Related Research* 2015; 473: 3564-72.

themselves, whereas the other half were randomized to make a treatment recommendation for a patient of their own age and gender.

Do you want to make a guess about the study results?

Surgeons were more likely to recommend surgery for another person than to choose the same surgery for themselves. They were also more confident deciding about their own care than making a decision for their patients.

Ha!

There you go — we've just been blatantly unmasked as *hypocrites*.

Under this premise, would you ever let someone else decide on your behalf whether you should undergo a surgical procedure?

Do you need another argument to support the principle of shared decision-making?

This fundamental concept entails building a true partnership between patients and surgeons. And this can only be achieved by incorporating patients' perspectives and personal values into decisions about the best treatment option, particularly in situations when there is no single correct medical answer available (you may remember from our previous discussion how often surgeons are confronted with uncertainty).

Interestingly, research in this rapidly evolving field has shown that well-informed patients who are engaged in their care tend to choose less invasive, less risky, and less costly treatment alternatives that are associated with better overall outcomes.[37] Shared decision-making has everything to do with empathy and compassion for our patients.

Let's face it: even if you're not empathetic and exclusively driven by *Funktionslust* and financial gains, you should still care about involving your patients in the decision-making for their surgical care.

---

[37] Page A. Safety in surgery: the role of shared decision-making. *Patient Safety in Surgery* 2015; 9: 24.

You're asking why?

Well, because studies have shown over and over again that effective communication with patients is associated with a decreased incidence of legal claims and lawsuits, better clinical outcomes, improved patient compliance with recommended treatment regimens, decreased unplanned readmission rates, and an improved perception by patients about the quality of care received.

If you're not already on the bus, now's the time to get on board.

Clearly, the historic 'paternalistic' care model is outdated and must be replaced by a modern collaborative team approach.

Our patients have an intrinsic right to speak up. And what we hear them saying today is: "Nothing about me, without me!"

Have you ever realized that your patient is typically the last person to know what's going on related to their medical care? We make all these decisions at rounds, team meetings, and behind closed doors in our offices. We simply assume that the patient will eventually know.

Have you heard the ominous anecdotes of hospitalized patients who called the hospital's operator to inquire about their diagnosis and discharge plans, because the rounding physicians never told them? Quite mind-boggling, to say the least.

Clearly, the success of a strong patient-surgeon partnership is based on mutual trust, respect, full transparency, and joint decision-making in all relevant treatment aspects.

So what's my own trick for knowing whether I successfully practice shared decision-making? I know that I've succeeded every time I leave a lengthy face-to-face conversation with one of my patients. Typically one involving multiple tools and aids, bone models, radiographs, and drawings. One of those conversations that last at least 20 to 30 minutes or more.

I am regularly astonished when the patient ultimately answers: "You know, Doc, I really wanted surgery when I came here, but after everything you told me I'd rather proceed with the non-operative option."

Whenever that happens, I get chills down my spine. I would then secretly tear up the add-on sheet for surgery that I had pre-populated (in the wrong assumption that the patient would opt for surgery after our discussion), and leave the patient's room with a huge smile on my face.

Why would I smile?

Because I know in that very instant, for the blink of an eye, I was probably the world's most effective "shared decision-making expert".

In those moments I know that my conversation made a difference in a patient's life — whether my hospital administrators like it or not.

By the way, I recently saw a provocative editorial in the renowned medical journal *JAMA Internal Medicine*. The article claims that disregarding patients' preferences for treatment decisions should be considered malpractice.[38] I would assume that everyone who read Michael Skolnik's horrifying story will second that proposition in a heartbeat.

[38] Allison TA, Sudore RL. Disregard of patients' preferences is a medical error. *JAMA Internal Medicine* 2013; 173: 787.

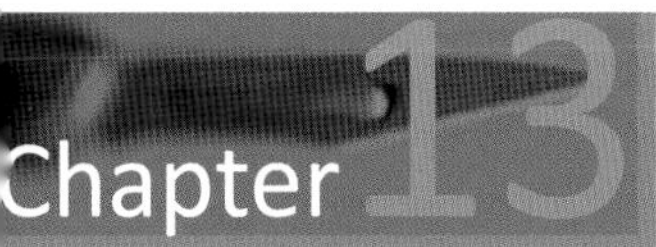

Patient advocacy: it's a team approach

"It's amazing how much you can accomplish when it doesn't matter who gets the credit."

Harry S. Truman (1884-1972)

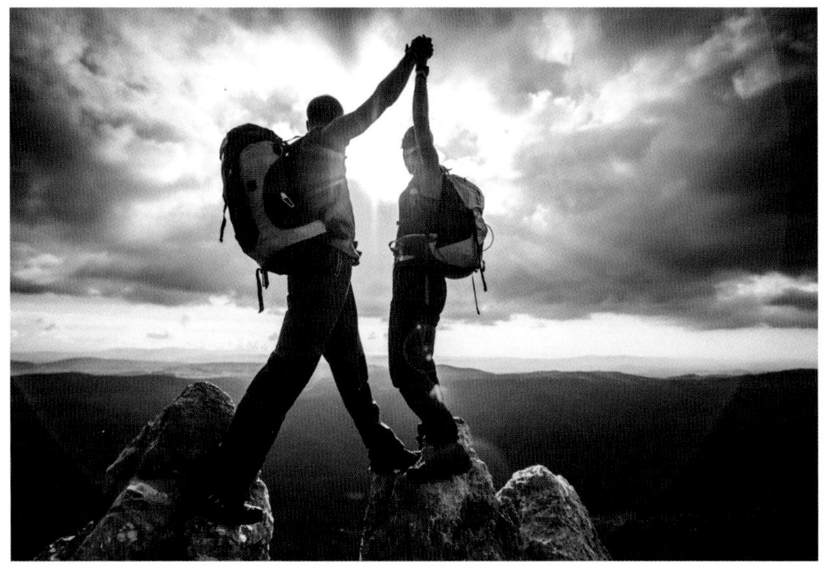

In the preceding chapters, I discussed the multiple responsibilities and duties surgeons have, to provide infallible, high-quality patient care.

What about patients' responsibilities?

Tough question, I know.

If I had to narrow it down to a simple imperative, I'd argue that it's the patients' responsibility to advocate for their own health, to engage in critical discussions with the care team, to challenge their surgeon with unanswered questions and concerns, and to proactively engage in the postoperative recovery and rehabilitation phase.

Maybe that sounds like a lot.

I don't think it is.

And while this might sound compelling and straightforward, bringing patients to that same realization isn't easy.

Consider the multiplicity of barriers we impose on our patients. Chief among them is our inability to listen. Remember our habit of interrupting our patients after just *12 seconds*, as previously discussed? This is especially egregious considering that patients who have to discuss the need for surgery are extremely vulnerable and exposed.

The 'white coat factor' comes into play here, too. Multiple studies have shown that most patients are reluctant to distrust or question their surgeon's advice, even if their own intuition suggests that something isn't quite right.

Just as Michael Skolnik signed his surgical consent under the influence of pain medication and time pressure, surveys have shown that many patients are frightened and feel pressured or coerced into having procedures performed that they didn't feel necessary.

Most patients are too reserved and intimidated to ask for a second opinion. They feel that such a request may insult the surgeon and irreversibly breach the patient-surgeon relationship. They'd rather have the surgeon like them than risk losing that rapport. This is analogous to the situation when you're unhappy about the quality of your food served in a restaurant, and yet, you're too intimidated to speak up for the fear of breaching your relationship with the chef. After all, this is the guy who's in control of covertly spitting on your undercooked steak prior to the revised serving.

A large-scale community survey among more than 10,000 patients in 12 metropolitan areas in the United States revealed that the standard quality of care indicators were met in just 59.4% of all patients.[39] This means that you could almost flip a coin to determine if you will receive appropriate care for standard screening tests, counseling and follow-up, and coherent medical treatment and surgical care for frequent surgical conditions.

If patients are too intimidated to question their surgical indications, how do they bring up the willpower to request a second opinion?

The answer is, they don't.

There is an imperative for change: patients need a different vantage point. Patients need a strong representative. They need an unwavering patient advocate who will fight the righteous cause on their behalf. A meticulous investigator who will ask all the tough questions that patients would not ask for themselves. Someone who will say: "Show me the data, doctor! What's your complication rate? How do you know? What are alternative treatment options? Who would you recommend for us to see for a second opinion?"

Wow!

How great would that be?

39 McGlynn EA, *et al.* The quality of health care delivered to adults in the United States. *New England Journal of Medicine* 2003; 348: 2635-45.

For those privileged patients who have a personal advocate, that person is typically a close family member. However, not everyone's spouses or partners necessarily possess the backbone, stature, and endurance to take on the conflict. They may feel as vulnerable and intimidated as their loved one. Just look at the horrible fate of the Skolniks. They lost their son Michael because they were too overwhelmed to question the surgeon's indication for immediate "life-saving" surgery. I know that Patty regrets to this day that she was too naïve at the time to consider confronting the surgeon with unanswered questions. After Michael's death, the Skolniks turned into uncompromising patient advocates for anyone else who needed their support.

So, if patients in general can't advocate for themselves, and their closest family member may be too emotionally engaged to think straight, who will take over this noble cause?

The answer is simple: anyone who is willing to step in for you. Even a complete stranger.

My friend Marc Pinto is one of these anonymous fighters for the righteous cause. Marc has an impressive personal history. For many years he worked like a madman as a successful consultant with Arthur Andersen. Later he was the CFO of a start-up venture and then the president of a real estate company. Eventually, he'd had enough and retired in his mid-forties.

Yeah, *mid-forties*. Pretty cool, huh?

When I say retire, I don't mean he checked out. Rather, he picked up a new endeavor. His new mission was simple: to make a difference and to help those in need. Let's be honest: Marc is a great guy, but he's not that selfless. Whenever he isn't serving others who need his help, he loves to ski in Montana and scuba dive around the world.

What's life if it's not enjoyed?

I met Marc in early 2015. He presented to my office seeking a formal second opinion for recommended treatment by a different surgeon at another hospital. From the minute I shook his hand, I was extremely impressed by his 'no bullshit' attitude of seeking a second opinion. Marc had done all the necessary homework and understood his injury pattern in depth. He'd sustained a complex fracture around his knee after a skiing accident in Big Sky, Montana (the price of early retirement, I guess!). Instead of sitting back and letting me drive the meeting, Marc challenged me by discussing radiographs, including 3-D reconstructions of his knee. He threw selected articles and Google search printouts at me in the quest for the best surgical treatment concept.

I still remember the thoughts that went through my mind during that meeting: if every patient was as engaged in the advocacy for their own care, I could terminate my own patient safety work immediately! Mission accomplished.

I examined Marc's knee, spent 30 minutes face-to-face answering all his questions. Then, I confirmed that the initial surgical plan was pristine and that I had nothing more to offer. For some reason, Marc appeared to appreciate my straightforward style of communication (or maybe he sensed some intrinsic empathy?).

He asked: "Can you do my surgery better?"

I sat back, looked him straight in the eyes, and said, "No".

I explained that he'd be in good hands with his original surgeon.

"First of all," I said, "I strongly applaud your proactive approach for seeking a second opinion. Most patients never do that, unfortunately. However, when the second opinion confirms that the plan of your 'first opinion' is perfect, why would you consider changing? If you were piloting a plane from Frankfurt to Denver, why would you enforce a deviated landing in Greenland, when the instruments confirm that all systems are up and running? The main purpose of a second opinion is to ensure that the surgical plan is coherent. That's exactly the service I provided today."

Marc understood, proceeded to have the surgery done at the other hospital, and had a rapid and uneventful postoperative recovery, without complications.

Just as it should be.

As impressed as I was about Marc's advocacy for his own health care, I was simply speechless to hear about his engagement for other patients in need. I learned about Marc's adventures when we chatted over dinner a couple of months after his injury.

I was amazed that Marc would travel around the globe to seek the ultimate medical care, cutting-edge trials, and top ranked hospitals and surgeons. Not just for family and friends, but even for near strangers like Suzie.

I'll let Marc tell Suzie's story in his own words (Table 6).

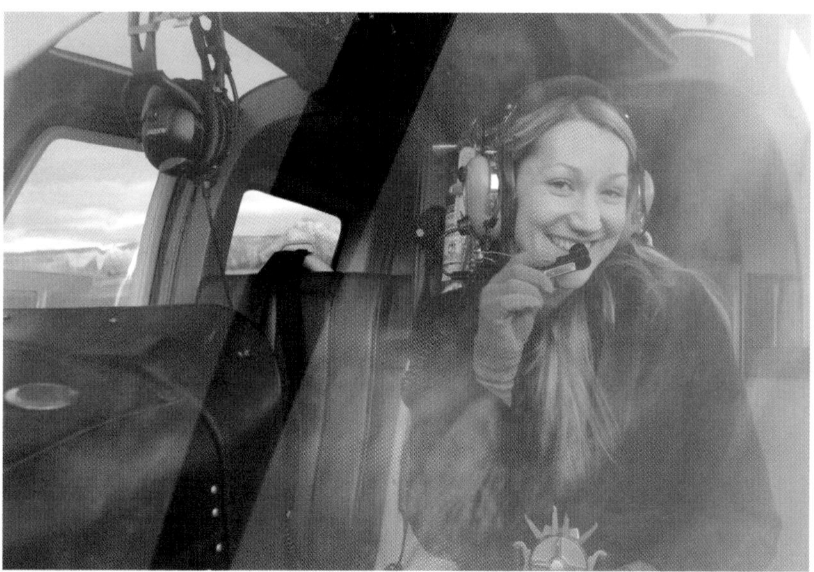

Suzannah "Suzie" Davis Ingraham (December 10, 1977 – July 3, 2010). This picture was taken on Suzie's 32nd birthday on December 10, 2009, in Sedona, Arizona, her favorite escape from 'Cancerland'. Suzie died 7 months later from terminal metastatic cancer. (Photograph provided courtesy of Marc Pinto.)

Table 6. Suzie's story.

It was February 2009, and I still remember where I was when I got an email from my friend Shane. His email was sent to a group of his friends, informing all of us that his longtime partner Suzie's cancer was back after 8 years. It had returned with a vengeance, with tumors in multiple locations throughout her body. I had known Shane for 2 years at that time. He managed a local scuba shop we frequent, and we had become friends. My partner Kristin and I had only had dinner once with Shane and Suzie, and before getting Shane's email I was unaware that Suzie had a history of cancer.

Eight years earlier, she apparently had a melanoma removed from her chest. At that time, the initial margins were not clear, so they performed a second surgery with a wider margin. Suzie passed the traditional 5-year 'cancer-free' mark 3 years before Shane's email.

Even though I had only spent a couple of hours over dinner with Suzie, I felt a calling of sorts to help in some way. At that point in time, I didn't know Suzie well enough to consider myself qualified to provide a comforting level of emotional support (that would change over the ensuing months). I approached her with a different proposition: I volunteered to serve as her 'medical advocate', helping her navigate the complexities of the health care system, insurance issues, and perhaps most importantly, the myriad of non-conventional alternative therapies available to a person dealing with metastatic melanoma. I had recently retired at an early age and was prepared to devote as much time as the volunteer advocacy may require. Somewhat to my surprise — and much to my delight — Suzie accepted the offer. I didn't know that this would forever change my relationship with Suzie and with Shane, in both a dramatic and a highly positive manner.

At the time of Suzie's tumor recurrence, there were few mainstream, conventional and quite draconian treatment regimens for metastatic melanoma available. While not dispensing with those as possibilities, it was the sense of the three of us that if there were an answer, it layed somewhere beyond the limited available care. So I began researching alternative treatments, clinical trials, and adjuvant therapies. Suzie's journey by 'melanoma time standards' was indeed very long and courageous. A number of selected episodes stand out as worthy of recounting; some to share a glimpse of Suzie's humanitarian spirit, some to share a glimpse of the presence (and in one case, the complete absence) of humanity by some medical professionals we dealt with. Finally, some anecdotes simply allow to underline the benefit of patients having a "medical advocate".

(1) "Wouldn't it be ironic..." We are fortunate enough to have access to a private plane, and at the time owned a place in Sedona, Arizona. So on Suzie's birthday, following a meeting with her surgeon to discuss one of her many surgical procedures, we surprised her with a blindfolded abduction to the airport, and whisked her to Sedona, far away from 'Cancerland' (Suzie's term for Denver). As we approached Sedona airport at night, the pilots informed us that there was a problem with the landing gear, and that we'd need to divert to a nearby alternative airport. Shane and I were mildly concerned, yet Suzie was the calm one among us, taking time to point out the extreme irony of a small-plane accident potentially beating the odds of her cancer fate.

(2) Medical allergies. Suzie was allergic to several medicines. She had been in and out of the hospital over a period of months. One or both of her parents were typically there during the days while Shane was working, and Shane stayed with Suzie at night. As nurses (and particularly unfamiliar ones) came in to administer medicines, Shane would always ask what was being administered. On three separate occasions, a nurse would have given Suzie a medicine to which she was allergic, were it not for Shane's vigilance and intervention.

(3) The search for clinical trials. Clinical trials seemed to be our best hope of prolonging Suzie's life, and ultimately her quality of life. We never openly talked as a group about her prognosis in terms of months, but we all understood the gravity of the situation. At one point, a member of Suzie's local oncological team had mentioned an upcoming trial that seemed promising. After prolonged waiting and repeated follow-up inquiries, the oncologist told us that trial participation was completely booked out. I found it hard to believe that there would not be one single trial slot open in the entire nation. So I began investigating. Knowing the designation of the trial and access number, it took me less than half an hour of an internet search to come up with the drug company and its list of trial locations (roughly a dozen), as well as the lead physician at each location. Armed with that information, I began searching for the individual email addresses of those dozen doctors. I ultimately learned that if I could find an article by one of them on the internet, the citation would include their email address if they were first authors on the publication. So after a half day of further dedication to internet research, I prided myself to have successfully retrieved the dozen individual email addresses. I sent the identical email to all investigators, briefly explaining Suzie's situation and asking whether they had any openings in their trial. The vast majority of doctors personally replied to my email, and it turned out that there were indeed three slots available in the United States.

(4) The search for the guru. About 9 months into Suzie's journey, it became apparent that a seemingly promising new melanoma drug (ipilimumab) was just appearing on the market and might hold a new promise for Suzie. Again, some protracted internet research led me to a specific doctor at Boston's Mass General Hospital who appeared to be the 'ipi' guru. Some additional research revealed his email address. He turned out to be a wonderful human being and a tremendous help as we navigated Suzie through the 'ipi' path. We regularly exchanged emails, and he was invariably prompt in responding to my questions and pointing us in the right direction. So while we were in Denver (and he was half a country away on the East coast) we managed to get a leading expert in the field directly involved in Suzie's care. Essentially by just tracking him down and asking for help. Nothing more complicated than that.

(5) The butterfly book. Two things became clear early in Suzie's journey: (a) her care would come from more than just one doctor, one hospital or even one city; and (b) she would have to undergo a myriad of lab tests and diagnostic procedures.

For some reason, getting complete copies of test results (particularly radiological tests, including a copy of the disk and the written report) is more complicated and time consuming than it should be. And metastatic melanoma appeared to be a disease not willing to wait for anyone or anything.

We would be regularly asked by a new medical professional for copies of prior test results. Early in Suzie's journey, gathering that information seemed to regularly delay progress. So I embarked on an important — yet exceptionally ministerial — mission of gathering all of Suzie's test results back to the time when metastases initially surfaced. I incorporated all data into a series of bound volumes, separated by identifying tabs. Suzie loved butterflies, so the cover of the first volume had her name, the date range of the tests, and a picture of a beautiful large colorful butterfly. When I delivered copies of that volume to Shane and Suzie at one of our breakfast meetings, she beamed with pride at having a 'book' about her, despite the troubling nature of its content.

(6) "A long run..." One path in Suzie's journey sent the three of us to the renowned National Institutes of Health (NIH) in Bethesda, Maryland. Suzie was being evaluated for admission into one of the NIH trials. After reviewing Suzie's most recent MRI, the experts shared their concern about a new tumor near her pancreas, and told us that for her to be admitted to the trial, she would first need to have that tumor removed. Its removal would involve a complex and very risky Whipple procedure. Suzie was determined not to give up, as the NIH trial seemed to hold the most promise. By now, she had her 'own' surgeon who had operated on her several times. Yet, we initially met with a local surgeon particularly experienced in Whipple procedures. He seemed puzzled why someone at Suzie's stage of her journey would be considering such an invasive surgery. We explained that this was an essential requirement as 'the price of admission' to the NIH trial which was our best hope. To our collective shock, the surgeon said he would not perform the procedure because of liability issues, and because — in his exact words — it was "a long run for a short slide". Whether he thought the surgery was indicated in the first place was certainly his call, but the incredible insensitivity with which he delivered the death message was outrageous and beyond belief. The "short slide" was of course what he deemed to be Suzie's remaining life expectancy, despite being completely uninformed, and apparently uninterested, in the details of the NIH trial (which was Suzie's last hope).

In the end, the melanoma metastasized to Suzie's brain and took her life within a short period of time. She died on July 3, 2010. But while none of us had talked about the number of 'months' she had left to live, Shane and I had been told at the outset that her prognosis was less than 9 months. Suzie lived for 18 months! That was twice the initial estimate, and most of it with a reasonably good quality of life. Shane and I realized that by taking a proactive role and not leaving a single stone unturned in the search for alternative treatments, we helped extend her life and her time with those she loved and had an impact upon. To this day, 5 years after Suzie's death, Shane and I remain the best of friends, with the strong bond of having shared an arduous and emotionally challenging experience as unwavering patient advocates.

Marc Pinto (July 2015)

Marc's impressive recollection of Suzie's story emphasizes that the sky is the limit for engaged patient advocates. This story also confirms why it is imperative for patients to find their own representative to steer them safely through the 'jungle' of the health care system.

It's truly a team approach.

"All for one, and one for all!"

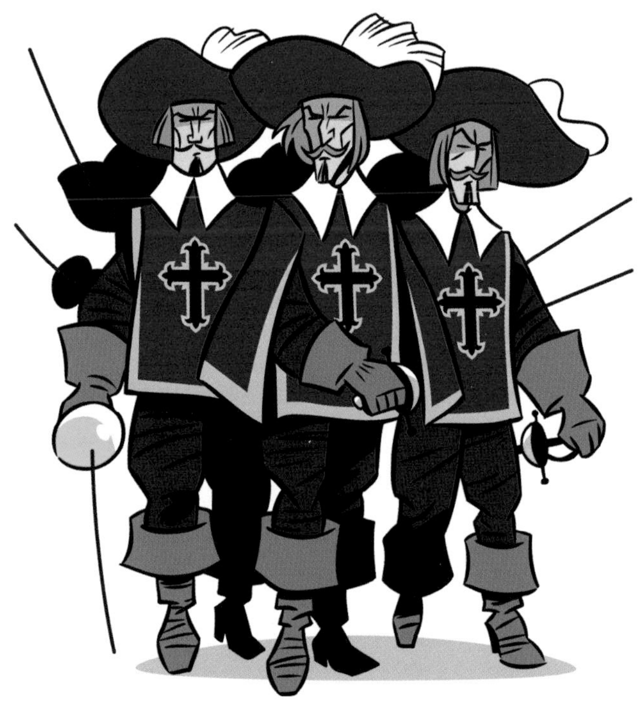

In 2015, the notion of a paternalistic 'omniscient' surgeon who unilaterally decides on his patient's best course of treatment has all but faded away under the shining light of the shared decision-making team approach.

By having a clear understanding of all treatment goals, expected outcomes, odds of complications and setbacks in the healing process, the patient-surgeon team can more safely navigate the dangerous waters of surgical care.

Obtaining a second opinion facilitates team building and establishes a strong mutual trust and credibility in the process. With the exception of acute life-saving or limb-saving surgery, most patients have enough time to seek a second opinion, either in person, remotely, or through their patient advocate.

There is no reason not to do it.

You don't buy the very first car you see at the dealership, right?

Let me be clear: there is no argument for a surgeon to ever be opposed to a second opinion. If the recommended course of action is justified, this will be confirmed by the second consulting surgeon. If not... well... then it's a good thing the patient requested a second opinion!

I want to share a final brief story about Marc with you; one that emphasizes the personal responsibility of patients to be proactively engaged in their own postoperative rehabilitation process.

Marc was just a few weeks out of a complex surgical procedure to restore the break around his left knee (a so-called "Moore type 5 bicondylar tibial plateau fracture-dislocation"). He wanted to change the pace during his recuperation by resuming his Indiana Jones-lifestyle and global adventure trips.

Marc was extremely meticulous and dedicated to full compliance in terms of weight-bearing precautions and knee range of motion exercises; certainly as much as any of our 'dream patients' ever would be (see the figure overleaf). His girlfriend Kristin even joked to me at dinner one night that she wished he'd be a little more lenient with his strict precautions after they go to bed at night...

	Reps	Hold	Sets	x/Day	X/week	M	Tu	W	Th	F	Sa	Su
Straight leg raise	10	3	2	6		✓	✓	✓	✓	✓	✓	✓
Quad set *Heel on bolster, push down knee*	20	5	1	6		✓	✓	✓	✓	✓	✓	✓
Seated short-arc quad *Hang leg and flex it from 0-60 degrees*	10	3	2	6		✓	✓	✓	✓	✓	✓	✓
Supine hip rotation *Heel on bolster, roll leg left and right*	20		1	1		✓	✓	✓	✓	✓	✓	✓
Four-way hip *Use walker, swing leg in all directions*	10		3	1		✓			✓	✓	✓	✓
Glute squeeze *Lie face down, lift knees off table*	10	5	2	1		✓	✓	✓	✓	✓	✓	✓
Bridges *Lie on my back, left leg in the air, straighten torso on bent right leg*	8	3	2	1		✓	✓	✓	✓	✓	✓	✓
Bathroom floor knee extension			3	2		✓		✓	✓	✓	✓	✓
Leg on shoulder *Lie on back, left leg on K's shoulder, push in all four directions*	10		2	1	4	NO		NO	✓	NO	✓	✓
Patellar mobilization	10		1	6	4	NO		NO	✓	NO	✓	✓
Modified side knee plank *Lie on right side, pillow between legs*	3	15		1	4	NO	✓	NO	✓	✓	✓	NO
Hip flexor stretch *Lie on back, lower left leg to stretch front of thigh*	3	30	1	1	4	✓	✓	NO	✓	NO	✓	NO
Braced march	10		3	2	4	II	NO	II	NO	II	II	NO
Side lying hip abduction *Lie on right side, raise left leg with glutes*	10	3	3	1	4	✓	NO	✓	NO	✓	NO	✓
Face-down lower-leg flexion/extension with resistance	10		2	1	4	✓	NO		NO	✓	NO	✓
Prone hip extension *Lie face down, engage core, lift leg–PROGRESS*	10	1	2	1	4	✓	NO	✓	NO	✓	NO	✓

Prototype of an engaged patient: Marc Pinto's personal 'rehab checklist' after his knee surgery.

Marc's mobility status progressed well. Around 6 weeks after surgery he decided to leave the preceding 'dark period' of anxiety and solitary confinement behind and he booked a trip to Crater Lake National Park in Oregon.

Traveling in a party of three couples, Marc understood that his own participation (on crutches) would somewhat limit the group's exploratory options. They methodically planned the trip to Crater Lake and patiently awaited a perfect weather forecast (somewhat, I imagine, analogous to D-Day preparations). When that day came, it was 73° and there wasn't a cloud in the sky.

After a scenic 2-hour trip, with Marc at the steering wheel of a rented SUV (as he had injured his left knee, he felt it was legitimate to drive with the right foot), they arrived at the fascinating Crater Lake. It became immediately apparent that a full view of the lake and its surroundings could only be obtained by climbing a snow bank, as there were no maintained viewing paths. Marc gently poked and prodded the footpath in the deep snow with one of his crutches, only to conclude that nothing good would come of this attempt.

As he never takes "no" for an answer, Marc started looking around for an alternative option. Sure enough, he spotted a wide sidewalk leading to a much smaller snow bank, atop which other tourists were taking in their full view of the lake. His intuition led him to drive the rented SUV up onto the sidewalk. One of the tourists was apparently aware of Marc's handicap and kindly guided him driving the SUV uphill. While this was clearly in violation of numerous National Park rules and regulations, Marc was committed. He was able to get the front wheels out onto the snow bank and then used the car as a 'railing' to pull himself up to the top.

Finally, Marc was able to savor the entire gorgeous view, unfettered by any visual obstacles. His subsequent photo session was abruptly interrupted by a visibly upset (and armed) park ranger who walked up to Marc and demanded to know what the hell he was doing. Marc explained the necessity of the exceptional situation. The ranger appeared neither impressed nor empathetic in light of the large SUV driven off road in the middle of the National Park. Clearly annoyed, the ranger uttered a sentence that remains enigmatic to this day: "Just because you're on crutches doesn't mean you can go anywhere you'd like."

Of course it doesn't! Being restricted to crutches typically implies the exact opposite!

Kudos to Marc for advocating for his own health and fast-track rehabilitation. This anecdote reflects the notion that — even in the absence of a dedicated patient representative — you should never hesitate to advocate for your own health and quality of life.

No matter what the park ranger says...

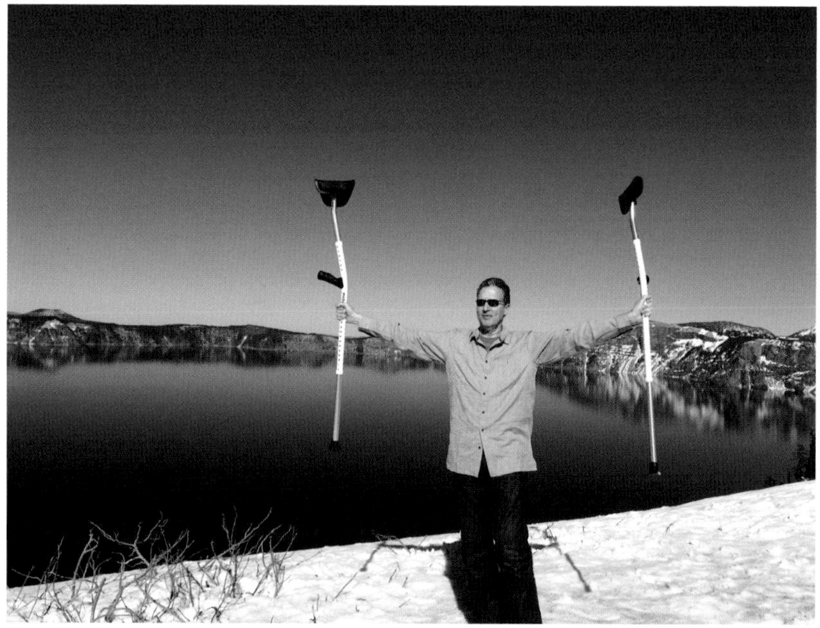

"Just because you're on crutches doesn't mean that you can go anywhere you'd like!"

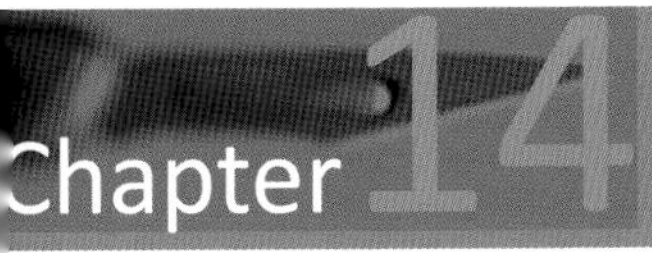

Questions a patient should ask their surgeon prior to surgery

"Does anybody have any questions for my answers?"
Henry Kissinger (*1923)

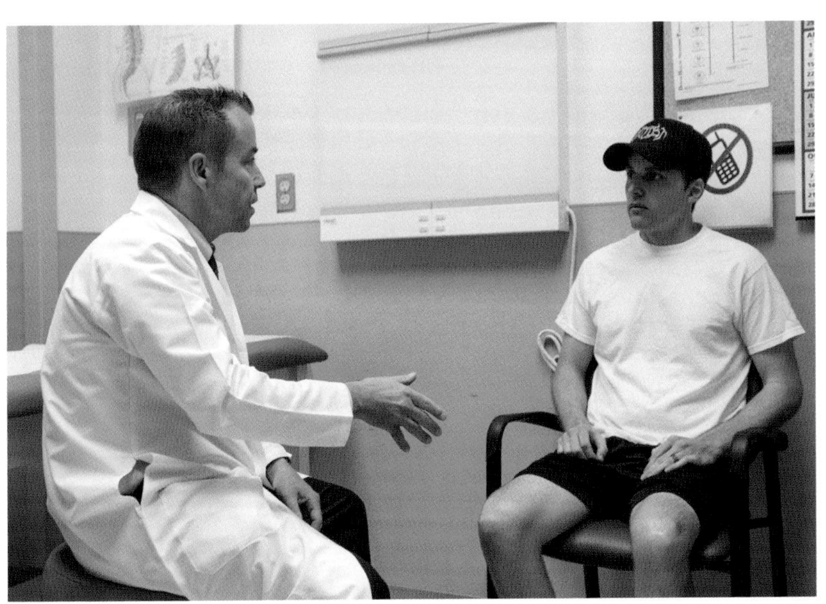

If you're reading this as a surgeon, I know what you're thinking: I can skip this chapter. It's exclusively targeted to patients, families, and their advocates, right?

Not so fast.

To the untrained eye, yes, that's what it looks like.

But the expert will easily recognize there's a 'hidden agenda' in this chapter; that is, to allow surgeons to foresee specific questions that might arise during pre-operative discussions with their patients. Taking it one step further, surgeons should consider proactively requesting patients to ask those important questions as a 'mandatory checklist' and a crucial part of the pre-operative decision-making.

Nice, right?

The truth is: patients are increasingly dissatisfied by the lack of meaningful participation in their own medical care and treatment choices. Instead of being asked to be involved in the design of their (surgical) care, most patients are interrogated via simple "yes/no checklists" in the pre-operative paperwork, for example, using standardized H&P forms.

Another truth: surgeons should be grateful to have fully engaged and informed patients.

Why? Because engaged patients can dramatically influence and improve the quality of their surgical outcomes. Just take another look at Marc Pinto's rehab checklist in the preceding chapter.

The key to being an engaged patient is to *speak up*. Remember how I postulated that a good surgeon should shut up and listen? In contrast, engaged patients must speak up. Patients should never be too shy, intimidated or complacent to advocate for their own health and to ask critical questions about the care they're about to receive. The quality of the pre-operative discussion with their surgeon may be the only chance for patients to stay safe!

In recent years, an internet-driven patient advocacy consumer movement has helped educate and empower patients to take shared responsibility for their health care.

You'd think this awareness would match daily reality.

And you'd be wrong.

I am still astonished how often my patients come across as obedient, submissive, uneducated, and unquestioning when it comes to asking questions about my recommendation to put a surgical knife to work on their bodies.

I recently returned from an off-site lecture trip and saw a patient listed on my OR schedule for a below-the-knee amputation. He was a very nice, homeless 62-year-old gentleman with severe frostbite on both feet. The patient had been seen and penciled in for a scheduled amputation by one of my fellows while I was out of town.

The pre-operative team was about to roll the patient back to the operating room when I stopped by to introduce myself to the patient. The man was ready to go and have his leg cut off. I put the brakes on it.

I explained to him the various available surgical salvage strategies we could use to attempt to preserve his leg. And then I asked him a simple question (that probably no one else had asked yet): "Don't you want to keep your leg?"

His eyes danced with joy.

"Yes, Doc! Thank you. I had no clue that saving my leg was an option!"

I cancelled the surgery and the patient was rolled back to the ward on my service. I consulted one of my microvascular partners who performed a plastic flap as a salvage procedure the next day. The patient's foot healed well and he actually walked out of the hospital 2 weeks later.

Unbelievable.

What went wrong? Why didn't the patient ask about other, less radical options? Why didn't he request a second opinion during the informed consent process with my fellow? Why was he so complacent in accepting the recommended dismembering and life-altering surgery?

This anecdote highlights just how crucial a patient's engagement as an active member of the care team is. It also doubles-down on the *conditio sine qua non* for the surgeon in charge to always go and personally see the patient. Had I not stopped by, this particular gentleman's fate would have been dramatically different.

Take away here, you better surgeons: never place a surgical indication without talking to the patient in person!

Situations like these can occur anywhere. Yet, I've found that teaching hospitals are the perfect breeding ground for lapses in care. In a setting where high-tech, state-of-the-art medical innovations are readily available, the personal aspects of medical care can easily be lost in translation.

Let me provide you with my personal checklist of *seven* specific questions that I recommend for patients to ask their surgeon prior to considering surgery (you can also consider this a 'cheat list' for surgeons).

1. Who are you?

If you are uncertain about the role and identity of the provider you're seeing, either in a physician's office or when you're admitted to the hospital, never hesitate to interrupt the discussion and ask: "And you are...?"

The person you consider to be your surgeon may, in fact, be (in ascending chain of command) a medical student, an intern, a resident at a varying level of training (the so-called "house staff"), or a fellow. Many times, patients are seen by physician assistants (PA) or nurse practitioners (NP) who support the surgical team (the so-called "midlevel providers").

Always ask to speak to your surgeon in person. Remember: in the hospital setting you'll have to ask to see the "attending" (in the USA) or the "consultant" surgeon (in the UK). This is the title for the most senior surgeon in charge of your medical care. Never accept an excuse for why you should not be able to personally speak with your surgeon in person.

No compromise.

No exception.

2. How clean are your hands?

You must be vigilant. Make sure your surgeon applies strict hand hygiene precautions before and after your encounter. The initial handshake provides a great opportunity to secretly peak at the quality of the surgeon's fingernails; are they trimmed and clean?

If not, you should rightfully question your surgeon's values and priorities related to your own safety in the process. (On a side note, always be suspicious of a surgeon who does not offer to shake your hand as part of the initial greeting.)

Does your surgeon appear to accept 'excuses' and 'exceptions' in such a crucial core safety measure as hand hygiene? When in doubt, ask the doctor to use the hand sanitizer — your life may depend on it.

3. Why surgery?

When the surgeon recommends for you to undergo a surgical procedure, ask why!

Ask if this is an 'absolute' or a 'relative' indication. An absolute indication means that there are no other meaningful non-surgical options available that can, ultimately, restore your health and quality of life. In contrast, a relative indication implies that surgery is not the only option, and that alternative treatment strategies should be considered.

The "why" should always be followed up with: "Or what?"

Ask the surgeon what will happen if you don't have surgery? What are the odds of improving your condition by fully committing to non-operative modalities, including pursuing a specific diet, regular exercise, physical therapy, or any other recommended strategy? Ask about the downsides and risks of non-surgical management. Ask about your expected short-term and long-term outcome.

Asking these key questions can greatly reduce your risk of suffering from a potentially unnecessary surgical procedure.

You should also specifically inquire about alternative surgical options, including less-invasive or minimally-invasive procedures. If such options are available, ask if they're part of your own surgeon's expertise. Should you possibly consider seeking care with a different surgeon, maybe at a different institution?

Challenge your surgeon with the question of who is considered to be the 'best' surgeon for the recommended procedure; locally, regionally, and nationally. Where would your surgeon seek care, or recommend family members and loved ones to have this procedure performed?

Ask about the case volume of this exact surgical procedure. How many cases has your surgeon done per week, per month, per year, and over an entire career?

Do the math to see if the numbers truly add up.

A dishonest answer may compromise your safety and quality of care.

4. What are the risks?

Remember, there is no such thing as a 'routine' procedure.

It is important that you inquire about the specific risks and complications related to a planned surgery. Ask the surgeon how he or she ranks your personal risk constellation related to age, body weight, pre-existing disorders, and medical history. If possible, obtain a copy of your previous medical records and have them available for your health care team to review.

Be sure to ask your surgeon about the risk of specific surgical complications, including the intra-operative injury to nerves, vessels, bowels, or other critical anatomic structures and organs in the proximity of the surgical dissection.

What happens if one of these structures is injured accidentally during the procedure? Is the surgeon qualified and competent to repair such a complication or would intra-operative help be required by a different surgeon or surgical team?

If so, is this expert help available in the same hospital? Is there a surgical intensive care unit available if required for postoperative monitoring?

Remember to inquire about the specific rehabilitation plan after surgery and the expectations related to the early postoperative phase (in or outside of the hospital), the expected level of pain and measures for pain control, restrictions related to mobility, diet and life style, permission to drive a car, expected return to work, expected short- and long-term outcomes, and potential residual restrictions and impairments.

I've often found that most disappointment and frustration stems from a lack of aligning clear expectations between surgeon and patient.

5. Who will perform the surgery?

If a decision is made to proceed with surgery, ask who will be the surgeon to physically perform the procedure. In a teaching hospital, residents in training or midlevel providers may be involved in most surgical procedures. Ask about their roles in your case. Will the attending surgeon personally 'scrub in' or just supervise the case from a distance (worst case: from his office)? These are reasonable questions that may make all the difference for the quality of your surgical care.

Don't be too shy to ask!

And don't let anyone wheel you back to the OR without personally speaking to your surgeon *face-to-face*.

6. Can I get a second opinion?

Ask your surgeon about the opportunity to obtain a second opinion.

(This is, of course, a trick question; "yes" is the only valid answer.)

If so, who to recommend as an established expert in the field, either at this hospital or elsewhere? Where would your surgeon go to have this specific procedure performed?

(Yes, this is another trick question: the answer should be identical to the one about the 'best' expert surgeon in the field.)

7. Why don't you listen to me?

Beware of surgeons who appear too busy to listen to your story.

Does your doctor take the time to sit down and talk to you at the same eye level? Does he/she check the clock while you're speaking? Do you get interrupted before finishing your sentence or question?

If the doctor interrupts you, resume your story from scratch: "Doc, I really need you to listen and understand my entire story."

Guess what? You can help your surgeon to become a better listener!

Remember that surgeons who appear to be poor listeners will likely also provide poor medical care. You should test your doctor's understanding of your story with provocative read-back questions, like: "Doc, how do you feel about the story I just told you? Which aspects of what I said do you feel are important to establishing my diagnosis and treatment plan?"

Does the surgeon thank you at the end of the appointment?

Do you feel heard and respected?

Make sure that there is always time dedicated to open questions at the end of the conversation. Don't get cornered with simple "yes/no" questions. Guide your surgeon to open-ended questions and elaborate on your story as you feel is imperative for the surgeon to fully understand.

You are in charge here; make sure you're getting what you need. I say, learn from our well-coached politicians on TV. Most politicians don't answer to "yes/no" questions, but rather find a smooth segue to turn to spotlight on their own story and agenda. This is the essence of Henry Kissinger's famous opening quote at the beginning of this chapter.

Tricky, but extremely helpful!

Let me finalize the main take-home points for your visit in the surgeon's office.

Remember that it's your personal obligation as a patient to come prepared to the appointment! Always bring your medication list and tell your surgeon exactly what medications you are taking; since when, in what dose, and at what intervals.

Highlight any allergies you might have and ensure the surgeon reads back and takes notes on the exact medications and allergies you listed. A surprising number of medication errors originate from vague and inaccurate medication lists in hospital systems. Take your time at home to write a list of specific questions, and make sure you get an answer to all questions before you leave the office. Talk to family members, friends, colleagues, and seek opinions from other health care providers in your own 'circle of trust'. If you have to, confront the surgeon with the questions or concerns raised by your patient advocates. Or, better yet, bring your strongest advocate with you to the appointment.

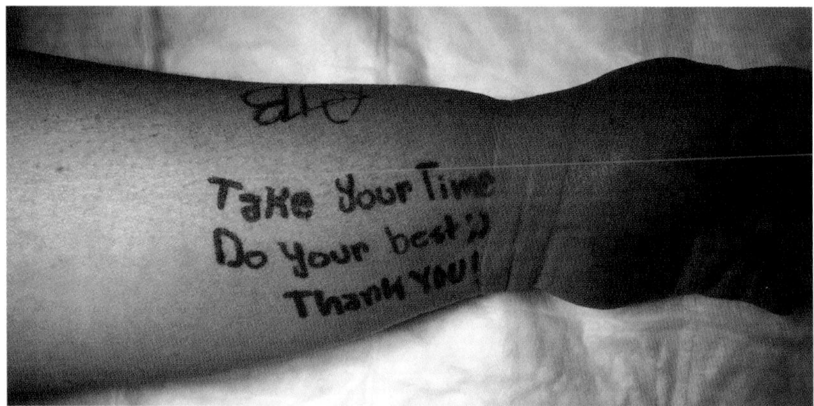

Anecdotal example of a proactive and uncompromising approach for patient advocacy 'in the trenches': this 45-year-old patient marked her own wrist with a personal message to the surgeon prior to undergoing elective carpal tunnel release on July 20, 2015. (Photograph provided courtesy of Kyros Ipaktchi, MD.)

If the decision is made that you will need surgery (with or without a second opinion), you should ask the surgeon all specific details about the procedure:

- "Will you personally perform the procedure? If not, who is going to do the surgery?"
- "Will there be assistants and trainees in the operating room?"
- "How long is the surgical incision and where will it be located?"
- "What are the general risks and potential complications associated with this procedure?"
- "What is your own complication rate related to this procedure? What is your own rate of surgical site infections?" (Be skeptical about a "standard" 1% to 2% answer.)
- "How do you know your complication rate?"

- "What is your reporting structure of complications and M&M process?"
- "Do you review *near miss* and *no harm* events?"
- "What scoring system do you use to grade your complications?"
- "What is your process of implementing action items to avoid future occurrence of identical complications?"

Don't leave your doctor's office without all questions answered. Never leave without knowing your specific diagnosis and treatment plan.

The least you should request is a current working diagnosis, especially if you require further diagnostic testing until a definitive diagnosis is established. You can't be rushed to surgery in the absence of a diagnosis, unless under life-threatening conditions.

If you're exposed to the potential risk of needing surgery, you clearly have nothing to lose.

Be honest.

Honesty is the key to every successful partnership. Make sure you answer your surgeon's questions with 100% accuracy and transparency. Don't try to look good by providing 'wishful thinking' answers. If you do, you may regret it later when things go wrong.

And trust me: things do go wrong.

In the United States alone, there are hundreds of thousands of preventable deaths from medical errors and surgical complications per year.[40] These numbers should provide sufficient testimony why you must strictly advocate for your own health.

No humility. No compromise.

You don't want to be the protagonist in Max Frisch's classic comedy *Biedermann und die Brandstifter* (1953) who handed over a pack of

[40] James JT. A new, evidence-based estimate of patient harms associated with hospital care. *Journal of Patient Safety* 2013; 9: 122-8.

matches to the arsonists in his own house, assuming that nothing bad would happen. When the going gets tough, you don't want to be an accomplice in your own downfall.

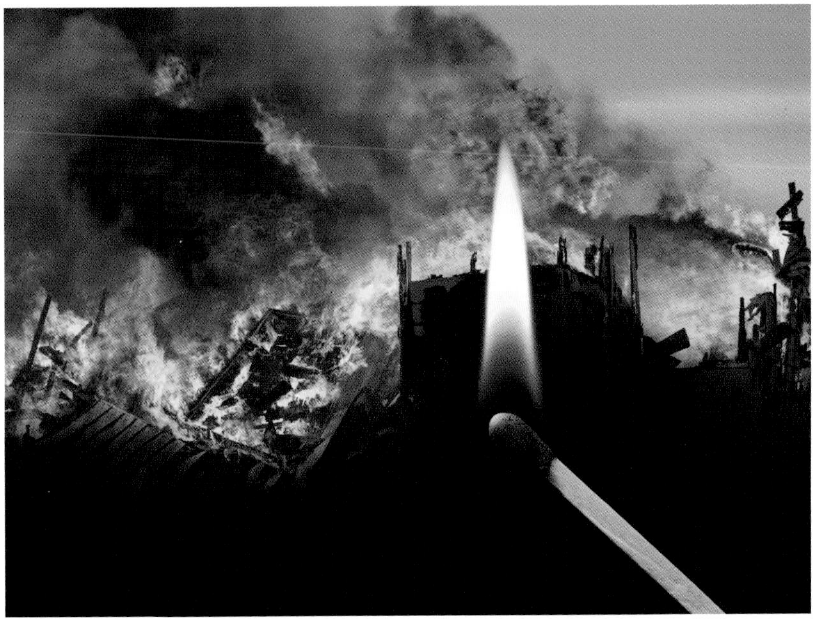

PART 4
The unsafe system

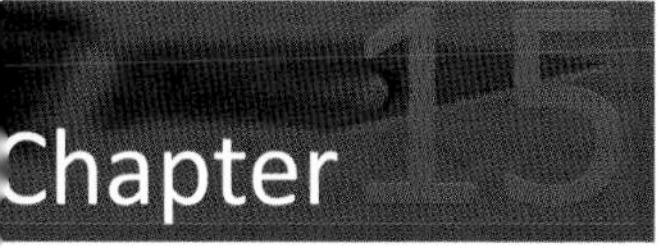

From 'blame & shame' to system failure

"Every surgeon carries within himself a small cemetery, where from time to time he goes to pray."

René Leriche, MD (1879-1955)

In the opening chapter of this book I told you about a patient who died on my watch when I was just an intern. It was traumatizing for me and tragic for the patient and his family.

I blamed myself at the time.

I still do.

But the truth is, in many ways, my patient was an indirect victim of the 'blame & shame' paradigm that dominated surgical training in the 1990s. And I regret to tell you that his death was, frankly, only the tip of the iceberg in terms of the horrible things I witnessed during my surgical training.

At the time, the guiding principle for resident education was the concept that with enough daily pressure, you can turn a lump of coal (a resident) into a diamond (an effective surgeon). Despite relentless pressure over years in training, it didn't take an expert jeweler's loupe to determine that the residents were as imperfect as fake gemstones.

We didn't have a diamond's shine. We had no brilliance.

Instead, the oppressive climate of reprimand, fear, and intimidation achieved the opposite effect: we became numb, tired, and indifferent to our patients' best interests.

There's a Chinese proverb that sums it perfectly: "He who is drowning does not fear the rain."

Want the honest truth? Our only goal was to save our own skins. And to do that, we turned into accomplices of a crooked system.

The list of ills was quite long. Patients were often unsafely discharged on the same day of the week that matched the Professor's ward rounds. The intent was to conceal bad patient outcomes and to avoid public scrutiny for poor-quality surgical performance. Similarly, critical patients in the intermediate care unit would receive a one-time 'jumbo' i.v. dose of Lasix® (furosemide) within minutes of the Professor's appearance on rounds. As any physician knows, this is a cheap (and potentially dangerous) trick to mimic the appearance of a 'peeing patient', one who had been sufficiently resuscitated to justify transfer to the regular floor — which means out of sight and responsibility for the rotating resident in charge.

These were ugly games, but not uncommon at the time.

Some readers who, like me, grew up in the era before digital imaging (PACS) will remember how their hospital's elevator shaft served as a silent testament to failed cases and undisclosed substandard care. This 'cemetery of shitty X-rays' would rise from the dead every other year when elevator maintenance workers found the stray films.

Gotta be kidding, right?

I wish I was.

I assume that most lay readers will be astonished by these revelations. At the same time, surgeons of my vintage will ashamedly smile, haunted by the ghosts of their own past ("been there, done that...").

Man, that was a rough time.

In Germany, the rules of engagement for junior residents were unambiguous, brief, and concise: "Haken und Schnauze halten!" (this extrapolates to "Hold the retractors and shut your mouth!").

Nice, right?

The thing is, the now historic concept of placing blame on individuals for failures neither trains us to be better surgeons, nor does it keep our patients safe. In fact, this actually puts our patients at a higher level of unnecessary risk.

There is a management philosophy that's been dubbed "just culture". It's designed to hold people appropriately accountable for their actions. And it is based on the presumption that blame alone is counterproductive and ineffective in mitigating risk and preventing harm; a 'no blame' approach to efficient oversight.

Now, 'no blame' doesn't mean that people shouldn't be held accountable for their actions; the important nuance here is that they should be held accountable *independent of the outcome* of their actions. Otherwise, individuals are simply blamed when things go wrong. And blame remains a pointless exercise. Identifying who's at fault neither solves the problem nor prevents a similar adverse occurrence in the future.

In contrast to the historic 'blame & shame' paradigm in surgery, the U.S. Federal Aviation Administration (FAA) has actually taken the opposite approach to ensure that commercial airplanes are safe. The FAA provides amnesty to anyone who admits having made a mistake.

Unthinkable!

This proactive program was designed to incentivize pilots and air traffic controllers to report poor personal conduct, including sleeping on duty or falsifying records. The FAA claims that since the implementation of the amnesty program, no other initiative has identified and fixed more local and systemic problems in aviation safety.

You're not surprised, are you?

Ironically, the current standards of compliance-mandated patient safety protocols originate from decades of work by lawyers and patient advocacy groups. Provocatively speaking, patient safety largely appears to represent a 'side effect' of defensive medicine and fear of medicolegal litigation. As physicians, we've been too complacent with the *status quo* for too long.

We should blame the lawmakers for this historic negligence; after all, surgeons have been rewarded for creating complications through financial incentives (by billing patients for another return to the OR) and prestige (by adding n+1 to your caseload).

Ouch.

That's a sharp one.

But it's got you thinking.

We'd never stand for lawyers directing air traffic controllers on how to avoid airplane collisions, right? We'd never consider using the 'blame & shame' approach in aviation safety? Can you imagine someone saying, "Well, the plane obviously crashed because the pilot is an incompetent idiot..."?

All the other high-risk industries outside of medicine (professional aviation, space aeronautics, nuclear plants and naval submarine technology, to name a few) have established redundant backup options that help mitigate errors before they occur. In engineering, 'redundancy' implies the duplicate or triplicate availability of critical components or system functions. For example, NASA endorses the fundamental principle of 'double-fail-safe' in all aspects of their high-risk enterprise. Yet, in surgery, errors in the care of our patients frequently lead to unintentional harm on the very first occurrence. We generally don't have redundant 'fail-safe' backup options. Most of us don't even dedicate a single thought to this important concept over the course of a surgical career.

Well, let's not give up too soon.

I have good news: it appears that over the past two decades, we've figured it all out. You'll be impressed to learn that we have successfully replaced the 'blame & shame' paradigm by a system that keeps our patients safe.

And everyone loves 'The System'.

Right?

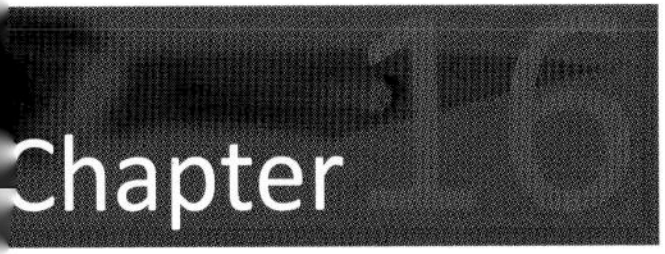

Why our current patient safety protocols are unsafe

"I will say that I cannot imagine any condition which could cause a ship to founder. I cannot conceive of any vital disaster happening to this vessel. Modern shipbuilding has gone beyond that."

Edward J. Smith (1850-1912)
Captain of the RMS Titanic

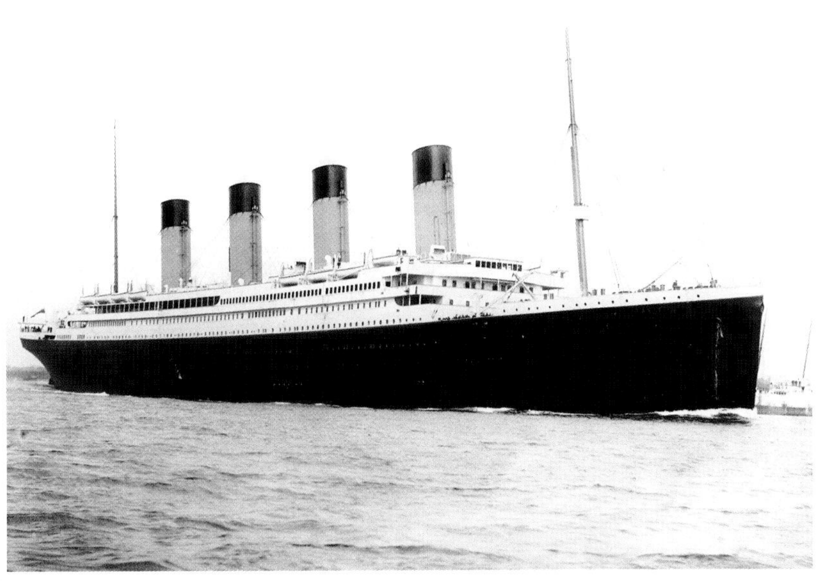

Today, systems-centered theories have largely replaced the now antiquated concepts of 'person-based' or 'blame-based' safety.[41]

Consider the RMS Titanic.

It used to be that captains took the blame if a ship hit an iceberg and sank. In the case of the Titanic, the tragedy was placed on the shoulders of Captain Edward J. Smith. Today, however, modern risk management strategies have all but eliminated the potential for human failure in contributing to maritime collisions.

Take a look at the sophisticated decision tree below (see the figure on the facing page).

Epic, right?

This algorithm was designed to help oil tankers avoid collisions and groundings.

Here's how this decision tree works: the probabilities of human error (circles) and the subsequent risk for downstream consequences that can ultimately lead to a ship collision are quantified by an underlying mathematical calculation at each step of the flowchart. Human factors represent the source of greatest uncertainty in risk management. Yet, quite impressively, this system for preventing maritime collisions appears to work; when was the last time you read about a ship collision in the news?

If only our system for preventing patient harm was as effective.

Or even as well thought out.

I'd like to take a brief look at "To Err is Human" by the Institute of Medicine (IOM).

I know, it's controversial.

---

[41] Holden RJ. People or systems? To blame is human. The fix is to engineer. *Professional Safety* 2009; 54: 34-41.

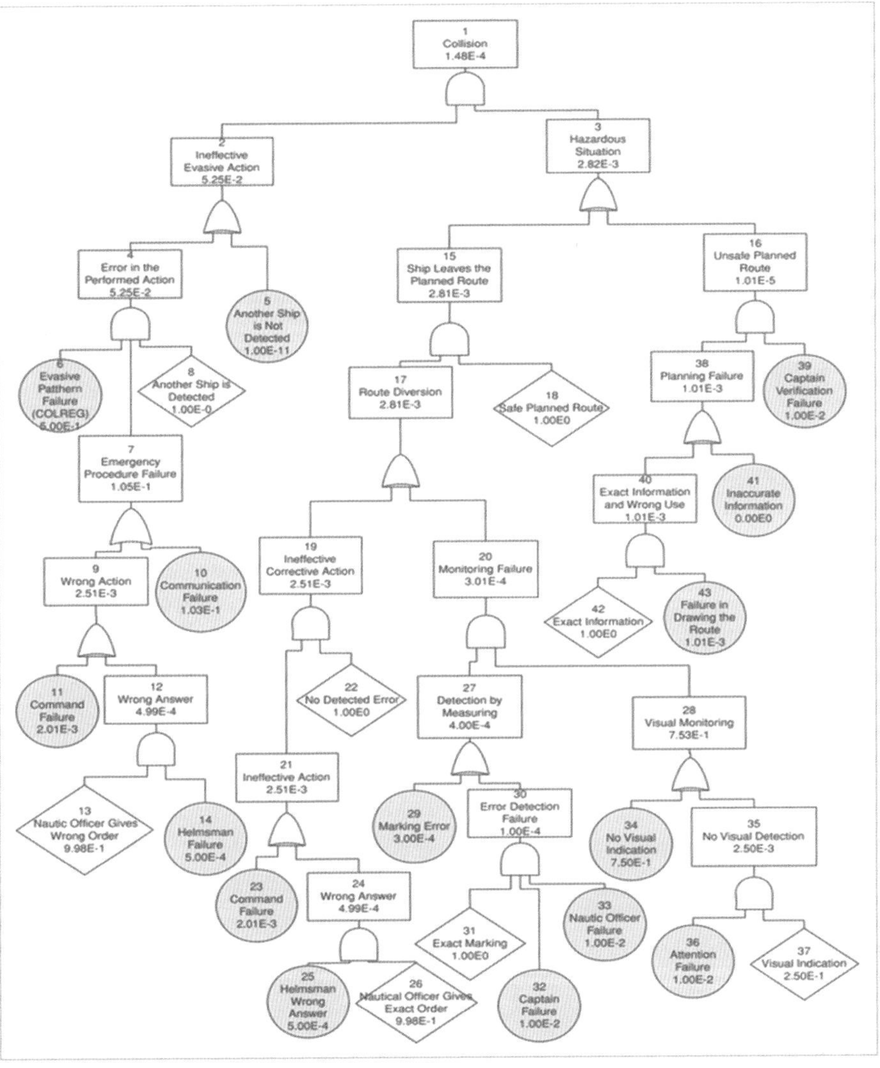

Human error contribution in collision and grounding of oil tankers. Reprinted with permission from: Martins MR, Maturana MC. Human error contribution in collision and grounding of oil tankers. *Risk Analysis* 2010; 30: 674-98. © John Wiley and Sons, 2010.

I also understand that you're probably sick to death of reading about the IOM report since it's been discussed *ad nauseam* for the past 15 years.

Just bear with me for a minute.

Seriously, it'll be worth your time.

For many, the IOM report is considered the 'kick-start' that launched us into the contemporary age of patient safety. When it came out (in 1999) the report estimated that at least 44,000 — and more likely up to 98,000 people — died each year in the United States as a result of medical error. It's difficult to underestimate the IOM report's 'shock and awe' effect. The result was an avalanche of new patient safety protocols and innovative safety checklists. With all that paperwork and new regulations, you might assume that systems-based safety protocols have reduced the rate of preventable deaths from medical error.

It's a valid assumption.

And it's totally wrong.

Why?

Well, I can show you.

Let's play a mind game and throw all the patient safety initiatives, national campaigns, regulatory compliance protocols, and safety checklists that originated in response to the IOM report into an imaginary black box (see the figure on the facing page). We'll label this box 'The System' (the one designed to protect our patients from unnecessary harm).

Then, we'll allow this system to work for 15 consecutive years.

Now imagine it's July 17, 2014.

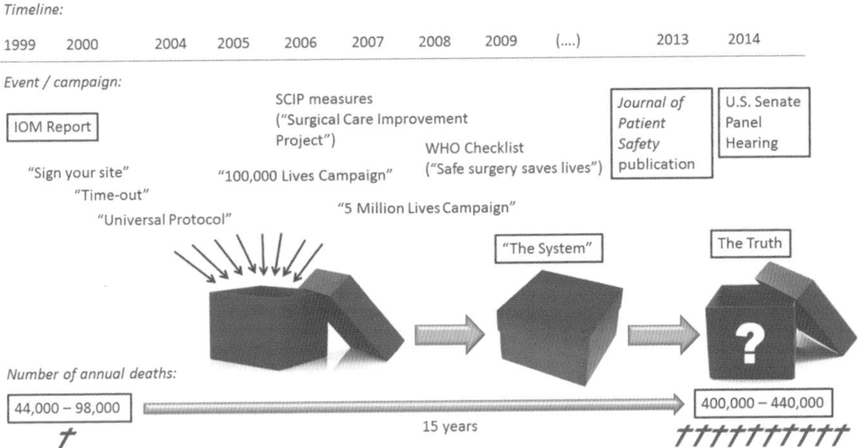

Fifteen years after the notorious IOM report.

Fifteen years after we shut the lid on the black box.

Fifteen years after we let the new system take control.

You're on Capitol Hill and you're eavesdropping on a Senate panel hearing about patient safety. There's a big emotional debate going on. Shouting matches left and right. In the midst of the ruckus, you hear distinguished experts and lawmakers claim that medical mistakes now represent the 3rd leading cause of death in the United States, and that only heart disease and cancer kill more Americans each year.

Hang on, you think, what about 'The System'?

Didn't the new system that we put in place put an end to this nightmare?

Well, let's look at the stats: current evidence-based analyses of medical error and patient safety data estimate that as many as 440,000 patients die from medical errors in U.S. hospitals every year.[42]

Yeah, six figures. And no, I didn't pull that number out of a hat.

What I'm telling you (and what the data show) is that 15 years after the IOM dropped its earth-shattering report, the number of patients who die from medical error has dramatically increased by five- to ten-fold.

Let me repeat that. It's gone up *five to ten times*.

And that's just the number of patients who die inside hospitals. The unreported incidence of patients who die at home (secondary to unsafe discharges, adverse effects from medications, and missed diagnoses) remains elusive.

So how is it possible that we have systems that keep us safe from nuclear reactor meltdowns, plane crashes, and maritime collisions, but we don't have one that keeps us from being accidentally killed inside a hospital?

Isn't a hospital supposed to be the *safest* place on earth, after all?

A few years ago, I decided to dig into this myself.

A good friend of mine, Ted Clarke, is the CEO of the largest physician malpractice insurance company in Colorado (COPIC). Ted is a respected senior surgeon and arguably one of the strongest and most pragmatic patient safety advocates I've ever met. For years, Ted and I have been meeting informally on Friday mornings in my office at Denver Health to discuss patient care issues and to brainstorm on new patient safety initiatives.

During one of these discussions, Ted let me know that COPIC has been collecting adverse event incident reports from more than 6,000 insured physicians in a prospective risk management database for several

---

[42] James JT. A new, evidence-based estimate of patient harms associated with hospital care. *Journal of Patient Safety* 2013; 9: 122-8.

years. This allows COPIC to recognize and resolve adverse occurrences with patients and their families in real time. It should be noted that COPIC's approach of early proactive resolution of adverse events (the so-called "3Rs" program, which stands for *recognize, respond, resolve*) has been shown to improve transparent communication and to decrease the number of lawsuits filed by affected patients.[43]

In the summer of 2007, Ted and I got to talking about the impact of the safety protocols and checklists that developed in the wake of the IOM report.

We spent a lot of that time discussing the "Universal Protocol" — a standardized checklist launched by the Joint Commission to avoid the accidental mix-up of patients undergoing invasive procedures and to prevent surgeons from unintentionally operating on the wrong body part.[44] Ted and I hypothesized that the mandatory roll-out of the checklist by all hospitals accredited by the Joint Commission should have led to a reduction in one of the most horrific preventable surgical complications; *wrong-site* and *wrong-patient* surgery.

Ted supported my request to perform a joint research project by getting me credentialed to query the vast COPIC database of more than 27,000 physician-reported adverse occurrences. After several months of retrieving and analyzing de-identified files during my off-hours work in the COPIC office, I was completely astonished by the findings.

You ready for this?

During a 6-year time-window that covers the period before and after roll-out of the "Universal Protocol" (July 1, 2004), there were a total of 25 patients who had received the wrong surgery due to a mix-up of their identities, and 107 patients who had the wrong (healthy) body part operated on (see the figure overleaf). What's most striking is that there was *no impact* whatsoever by the new system.

---

[43] Gallagher TH, *et al.* Disclosing harmful medical errors to patients. *New England Journal of Medicine* 2007; 356: 2713-9.

[44] Stahel PF, *et al.* The 5th anniversary of the "Universal Protocol": pitfalls and pearls revisited. *Patient Safety in Surgery* 2009; 3: 14.

No difference in the numbers.

Another blatant example of 'system failure'.

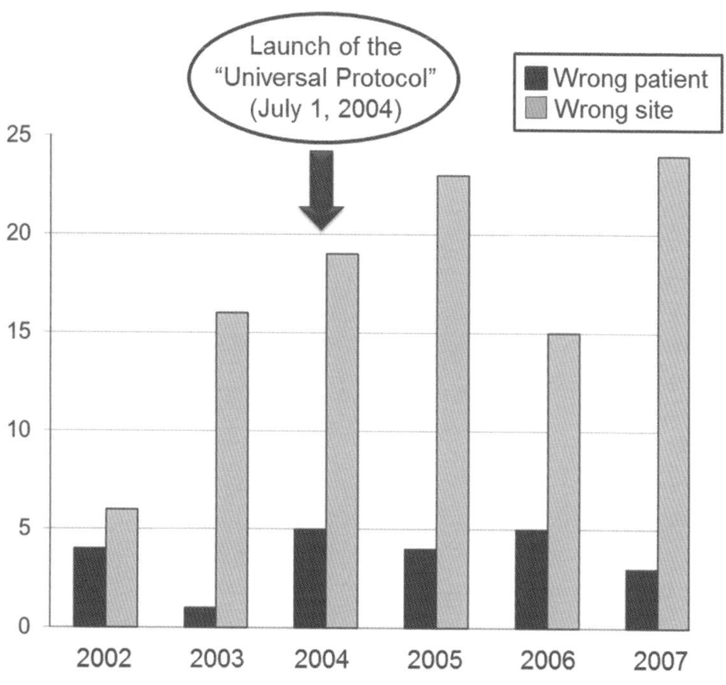

Wrong-patient and wrong-site surgery occurrences in Colorado before and after implementation of the "Universal Protocol" on July 1, 2014. Adapted with permission from: Stahel PF, *et al.* Wrong-site and wrong-patient procedures in the Universal Protocol era: analysis of a prospective database of physician self-reported occurrences. *Arch Surg* 2010; 145: 978-84. © American Medical Association, 2010.

Imagine for one second if you were one of these patients!

Most (if not all) people are anxious about having surgery. I imagine many toss and turn in the nights leading up to the operation even after understanding all the risks and benefits of having the procedure. And here they are putting on a brave face, convinced that you know what's best for them; only to come out of anesthesia to find you standing beside their bed, shamefully admitting you 'mixed them up' with another patient. Or that you accidently operated on their left side when you meant to operate on their right.

It's a mad-surgeon nightmare; the stuff of horror films.

In our COPIC study, a total of 43 patients sustained significant harm, and one patient died as a consequence of wrong-site surgery (see Table 7).

Table 7. Results from our study reflecting the extent of patient harm from wrong-patient and wrong-site surgical procedures. Reprinted with permission from: Stahel PF, *et al.* Wrong-site and wrong-patient procedures in the Universal Protocol era: analysis of a prospective database of physician self-reported occurrences. *Arch Surg* 2010; 145: 978-84. © American Medical Association, 2010.

	No. (%)	
Outcome	Wrong-patient cases (n=25)	Wrong-site cases (n=107)
Death	0	1 (0.9)
Significant harm or functional impairment	5 (20.0)	38 (35.5)
Minimal harm or functional impairment	8 (32.0)	65 (60.7)
No-harm event	9 (36.0)	3 (2.8)
Outcome equivocal or not determined	3 (12.0)	0

Part 4

Why?

Why on Earth does this happen?

How is it that pre-operative checklists fail to keep patients safe from preventable complications, dubbed as "never events" because they should *never* occur?

Recently, I read an interesting article in *The Wall Street Journal* that went into the problem of surgical "never events" and the failure of safety checklists.[45] The article claims that in the United States alone, surgeons leave unintentionally retained foreign objects (towels, sponges, instruments) inside a patient around 39 times a week, operate on the wrong patient around 20 times a week, and operate on the wrong location of the body around 20 times per week.

Mind-boggling!

Atul Gawande, the world-renowned patient safety 'guru', provides a compelling argument for the use of surgical safety checklists in his bestselling book dedicated to the topic.[46] He states:

> "In a complex environment, experts are up against two main difficulties. The first is the fallibility of human memory and attention, especially when it comes to mundane, routine matters that are easily overlooked under the strain of more pressing events. A further difficulty, just as insidious, is that people can lull themselves into skipping steps even when they remember them. Checklists seem to provide protection against such failures."

Obviously, checklists don't make a surgeon any smarter, more knowledgeable, better trained, or more technically skilled. But checklists do protect us from forgetting or skipping important steps in the 'heat of the action'.

---

[45] Landro L. How to Make Surgery Safer. *The Wall Street Journal*, February 17, 2015.

[46] Gawande A. *The Checklist Manifesto*. New York, USA: Metropolitan Books, 2009.

Anyone who's a fan of the classic film *Home Alone* (1990) will recall the dramatic consequences of a 'checklist failure'. It was an oversight during the family's hectic departure for a Christmas trip to Paris that left Kevin stranded at home. All hyperbole aside, this scenario is awfully close to a busy and distractive climate in the OR.

I will disclose to you that I'm a huge believer and advocate for checklists. In fact, I use them every day, in and outside of the hospital.

Need an example?

My brother-in-law Nate is a medical student in West Virginia. He regularly visits us in Colorado and stays at our house for a couple of months during the summer break. Normally, Nate parks his SUV in the driveway just outside our garage. When I leave to go to work early in the morning, I pull my Jeep out of the garage backwards. What do you think the chances are of my unintentionally hitting Nate's car?

It's certainly bound to happen, right?

Just think of the multiple early morning distractions. Between grabbing my laptop and papers while calling the OR bridge to coordinate my first case and ensuring not to spill my freshly brewed to-go cup of coffee as I walk out the door, my mind is all but focused. What are the chances that one of these mornings I'll forget that Nate parked behind me?

I'd argue that — per Murphy's Law — the probability is close to 100%. However, in the past 3 years, I have not backed into Nate's car once. Not even a ding.

How was I able to decrease risk from near 100% to zero? With a one-sentence checklist; a sticky note on my rear view mirror that simply states: "Dude, watch out for Nate's car!"

It took me a while to understand why some checklists work and others fail. I finally got it in the summer of 2010. And when it did, it hit me like lightning.

We were hosting our annual regional trauma conference in picturesque Breckenridge, Colorado. I was scheduled to give a keynote lecture entitled: "How to Prevent Wrong-Site Surgery" to a group of around 350 surgeons, emergency physicians, and OR personnel. As I stepped up to the podium, I challenged the audience with a provocative question: "How many of you have ever produced, witnessed, or heard of a wrong-site surgery in your own practice?"

I was met with complete silence.

Nobody moved. Nobody spoke. Nobody even raised a hand.

"That's what I expected! I'm speaking today on a topic that is completely irrelevant to everyone in this audience. We might as well just call it a day, right? Step outside into the conference lobby and I'll buy everyone a round of beers..."

There was an outbreak of subdued laughter.

I obviously proceeded giving my lecture as planned. The emphasis of my presentation touched on the imminent problem that wrong-site surgery is so exceedingly rare that we hardly ever take the risk into consideration in our busy practice. Clearly, most of us will never be confronted with such a horrible complication during an entire career. This mental pitfall is nicely exemplified in a quote by the creator of the famous "Swiss Cheese Model" of system errors, and author of the landmark book, *Human Error.*[47] James Reason said:

> "Accidents do not occur because people gamble and lose; they occur because people do not believe that the accident about to occur is at all possible."

Just Google a YouTube video of the 1986 Challenger disaster and you'll see this notion of incredulity manifest on the astonished faces of the CAPCOM flight controllers at mission control as they witness the Space Shuttle explosion on their monitors.

---

[47] Reason J. *Human Error.* Cambridge, UK: Cambridge University Press, 1990.

What happened to NASA's 'double-fail-safe' protocol?

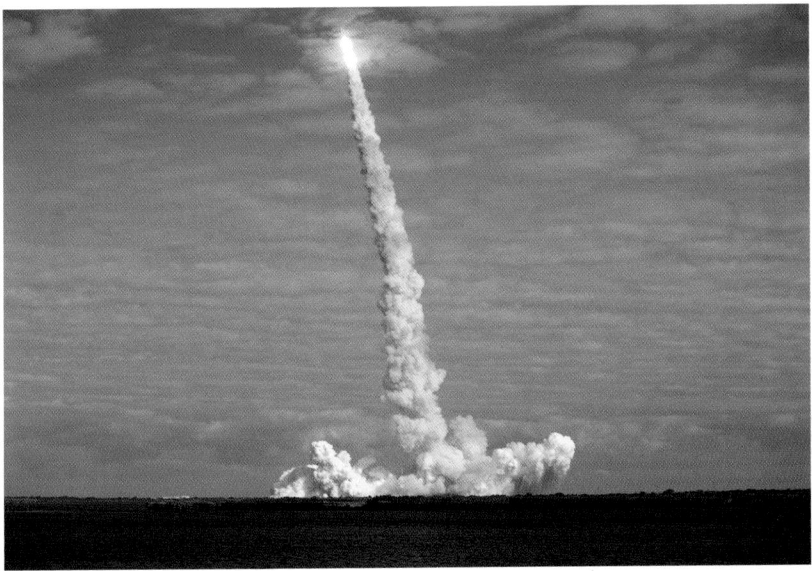

I would imagine that the extent of acute disbelief at the mission control center in Houston ("I never saw that coming!") is no different from that of any of the surgeons who performed the 107 wrong-site and 25 wrong-patient procedures in our study.

As I concluded my presentation in Breckenridge, I offered to answer questions. There were just a few generic questions and comments. Then, the audience dissolved for the coffee break. As I closed my laptop and wrapped up the power cable, a distraught gentleman in his mid-fifties walked up to the podium, shook my hand, and introduced himself. I remember being a bit annoyed as I saw my coffee break fade away due to this guy who might as well have asked his question during the preceding Q&A session. My initial irritation immediately switched to astonishment, however, as the man told me his story.

"Hi," he said, "My name is Jimmy Reed.[48] I've been a sports surgeon in private practice for more than 20 years. I really enjoyed your lecture. I am humiliated to admit that I have indeed committed a wrong-side surgery on a young patient several years ago. I accidentally operated on her wrong knee."

Wow, here it was in the flesh.

"Honestly," he continued, "I really wanted to raise my hand when you asked your introductory question, but I just couldn't do it. I was too ashamed to admit my failure in front of my peers."

I was speechless. Even more, I was about as ashamed as Jimmy. I'd never intended my 'attention-catcher' opening question to have such haunting personal ramifications. I felt like an idiot.

Jimmy continued: "You know, today, my orthopedic career is in ruins. I was sued and lost my license. Afterwards, my partners kicked me out of our practice. I stopped socializing with colleagues and then it got worse. I started drinking, and I eventually had to get counseling and therapy. I was admitted to rehab for a few weeks and my wife left me. We divorced a year later. I don't blame her; I must have turned into a miserable husband, and I was clearly no longer able to function as the head of our family."

I had no words.

My mouth was dry; my tongue stone. I knew that anything I'd say at that point would be completely out of place and irrelevant. So I just shut my mouth and kept listening.

"But the main reason I'm imposing on you is to give you a personal insight: when we performed our pre-operative 'time-out' and confirmed the wrong knee as the 'correct site' to be prepped and draped, there were seven other people in the operating room with me. Seven! None of

---

[48] Name changed to avoid any resemblance to actual individuals.

them noticed the dramatic error. None of them spoke up. None of them pulled the last-minute safety break prior to my skin incision. None of them stopped me from harming my patient and from ruining my life and career."

I nodded my understanding as Jimmy finished his story.

"You must never forget this part of it: checklists don't work if the team doesn't believe in them. Unless you've got complete buy-in, checklists can actually contribute to the risk of things going wrong. You see, they introduce an erroneous and dangerous sense of absolute security, a pure illusion of safety."

Jimmy turned around and left me standing alone on the podium of an empty lecture hall. I never saw the guy again.

What he had shared with me was the answer to my quest.

It isn't enough to be a better surgeon; we must be better leaders. We have to hold our entire team accountable for full compliance to surgical safety checklists.

That day, I pledged that I would never again accept a mediocre 'time-out' prior to a skin incision. There would be no joking or laughing in the OR during a checklist procedure. No distraction by anyone in the team.

From there on, it would be my personal obligation to consistently enforce a 'sterile cockpit' during the surgical time-out. This is a reference to the standardized, undisturbed cockpit during the takeoff and landing procedures aboard any commercial aircraft.

The sterile cockpit directive by the FAA requires pilots and the flight crew to refrain from any non-essential activities during critical phases of flight below 10,000 feet altitude.

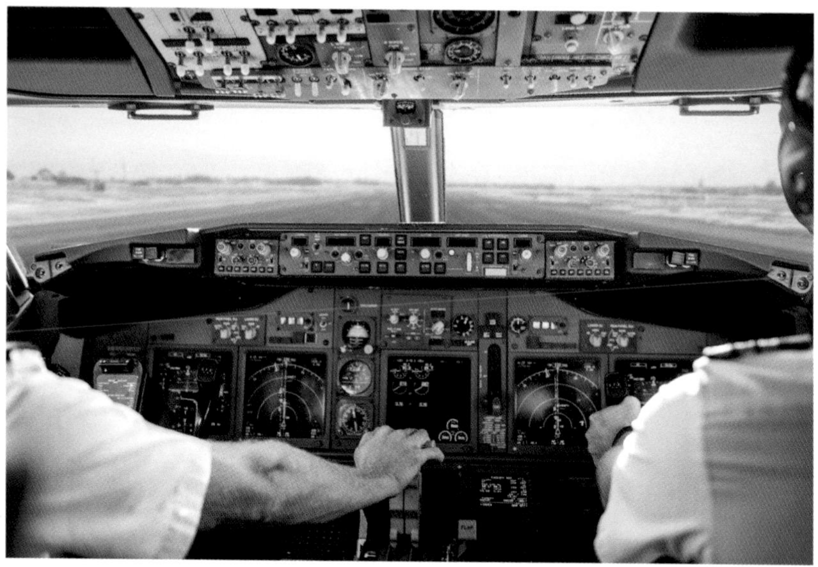

(This is why you hear that classic 'bling' sound that chimes after takeoff; it is a signal to the crew that the sterile cockpit 'time-out' is over once the plane reaches 10,000 feet.)

Take a minute to read the short and concise FAA regulation designed to define and enforce a sterile cockpit (U.S. FAR 121.542/135.100):

- No certificate holder shall require, nor may any flight crewmember perform, any duties during a critical phase of flight except those duties required for the safe operation of the aircraft. Duties such as company required calls made for such non-safety-related purposes as ordering galley supplies and confirming passenger connections, announcements made to passengers promoting the air carrier or pointing out sights of interest, and filling out company payroll and related records are not required for the safe operation of the aircraft.
- No flight crewmember may engage in, nor may any pilot in command permit, any activity during a critical phase of flight which could distract any flight crewmember from the performance of his or her duties or which could interfere in any way with the proper

conduct of those duties. Activities such as eating meals, engaging in non-essential conversations within the cockpit and non-essential communications between the cabin and cockpit crews, and reading publications not related to the proper conduct of the flight are not required for the safe operation of the aircraft.

- For the purposes of this section, critical phases of flight includes all ground operations involving taxi, takeoff and landing, and all other flight operations conducted below 10,000 feet, except cruise flight.

So the next time you call for a pre-operative 'time-out', keep a mental note to compare this strict FAA scenario with that of the 'pseudo-discipline' in the operating room (or the Christmas trip packing chaos in the movie *Home Alone* for that matter).

I'll never forget Jimmy Reed's words. They're my eternal admonition.

As I think back trying to understand why my own little 'sticky note checklist' has kept me 100% safe from accidentally bumping into Nate's car, the answer is now crystal clear: it's because I designed and implemented this checklist myself.

I own it.

I live it.

I respect it.

And I believe in it.

And nothing more and or less than that same level of commitment will keep our patients safe. It's time for us to start believing in our own safety checklists.

If we want to be credible leaders, it's our obligation to pass the same culture of discipline on to our team and to our trainees — the next generation of *better surgeons*.

Chapter 17 "See one, do one..." — no time to "teach one"

"True leaders don't create followers; they create more leaders."

Thomas J. (Tom) Peters (*1942)

Can I see the attending surgeon?
I'm not gonna play Guinea Pig for
some schmucks in training...
bigz

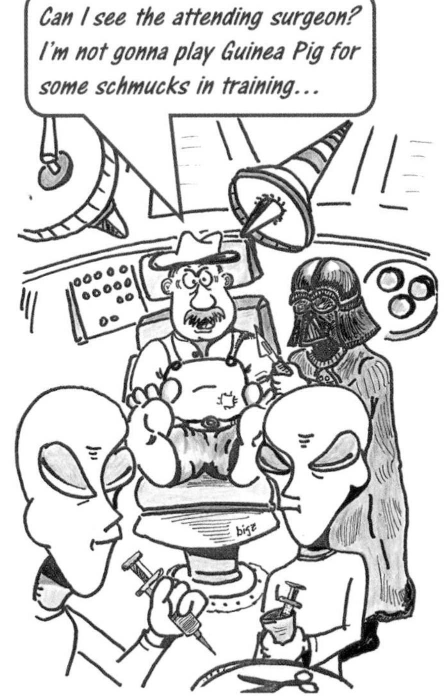

Let's finalize the 'system failure' discussion with another unrecognized problem that will have a dramatic impact on future generations of surgeons: work-hour restrictions that deprive our trainees of a coherent surgical experience, and breakdown in communication resulting from the multiplicity of subsequent handovers of care.

For this purpose, please allow me to take a minute to go back to the origins of my own surgical training.

I'll admit that for me, learning 'how to cut' took about twice as long as it should have.

Eleven years to be exact.

Yes, I know, I'm just a slow learner.

Considering that my current trainees at the University of Colorado graduate within just 5 years, I was very slow. Then again, surgical residency training programs on the other side of the pond are quite different from those in the States.[49]

The Accreditation Council for Graduate Medical Education (ACGME) tightly regulates American residency programs. In contrast, German residents are generally employed by hospitals through contracts of limited duration. And there is no guarantee of completing the surgical training at a particular institution. If the truth be told, the majority of residents have to go 'job hunting' to sustain their own training until graduation.

In Germany, the success and speed of surgical training is largely at the discretion of the department chairman. This historic (and unquestionably antiquated) system doesn't even ensure a resident will actually graduate from training to become a board-certified surgeon.

Looking back, I still remember the oldest resident I'd ever met in Germany: Gerhard Weidenfeller[50] was a grumpy old man with a long

---

[49] Stahel PF, Flierl MA. Orthopedic residency training in Germany: an endangered species? *Orthopedics* 2008; 31: 742-3.

[50] Name changed to avoid any resemblance to actual individuals.

white moustache he'd grown over more than 30 years of miserable residency training. And for Gerhard, there was no end in sight. Believe it or not: "Assistenzarzt Weidenfeller" was 62 years old (and close to retirement!) when I worked with him in Berlin.

Let me just hammer that home again: he'd been a resident for 35 years!

Yet, regardless of the vast differences in surgical training between Germany and the United States, both systems are actually facing the same major challenge in the 21st century: *resident work-hour restrictions.*

Here, it's worth taking a minute to look back at the evolution of how resident work-hour restrictions came to be and why I consider this another new 'system' of questionable efficacy.

It all started with the widely publicized death of an 18-year-old college freshman, Libby Zion, in 1984. Libby's death was attributed to gross negligence in the ED of a teaching hospital in New York. And the blame fell on the two young (PGY-1 and PGY-2) residents responsible for Libby's care after her admission for flu-like symptoms.

The subsequent investigation of Libby's preventable death revealed inadequate staffing and resident fatigue as the main contributing factors. In response, New York State adopted the Libby Zion Law in 1989. It's a regulation that limits resident physicians' work in New York State hospitals to 80 hours per week and to 24 hours of consecutive work. In 2003, the ACGME adopted similar regulations for all accredited medical training institutions in the United States.

These rules still apply today.

At first glance, it makes sense that a patient would want to be operated on by a surgeon who is wide-awake and well rested. In fact, a provocative study published in *Nature* in the 1990s showed that a single night of sleep deprivation is equivalent to being drunk.[51] In this study, the temporal decrease in cognitive psychomotor function in 40 volunteers was the

---

[51] Dawson D, Reid K. Fatigue, alcohol and performance impairment. *Nature* 1997; 388: 235.

Part 4

same, independent of whether the participants stayed awake for 28 consecutive hours or drank 10-15g alcohol every 30 minutes until their blood alcohol level reached 0.1% (see the graphs below).

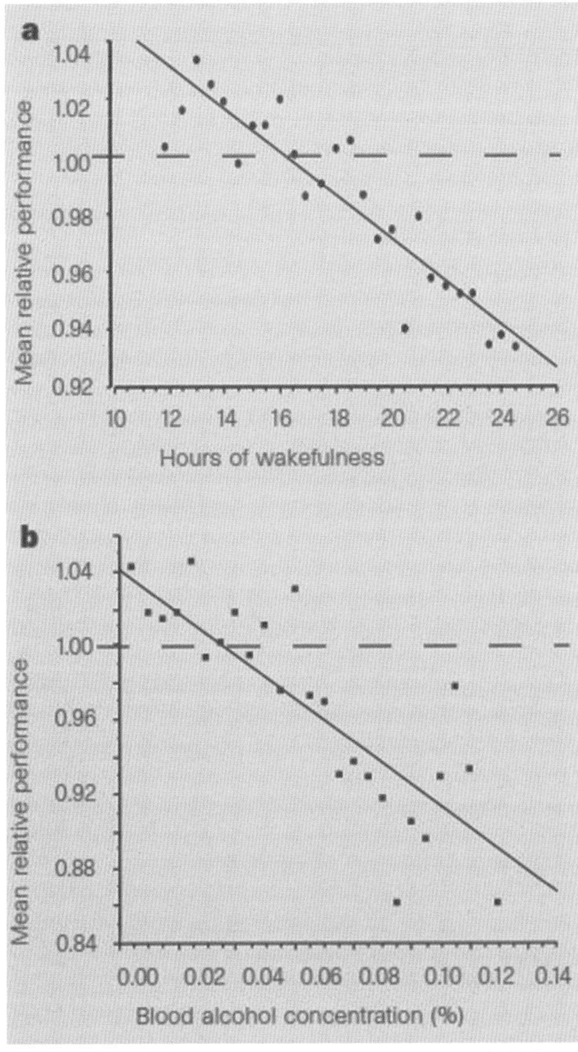

Reprinted with permission from: Dawson D, Reid K. Fatigue, alcohol and performance impairment. *Nature* 1997; 388: 235. © Nature Publishing Group, 1997.

Damn!

That's impressive stuff, right?

Subsequent research corroborated the same hypothesis – sleep deprivation impairs clinical performance.[52] These studies were ultimately the 'tipping point' in the drive for a change in ACGME regulations implemented in 2003.

Again, it makes sense.

Or does it?

Do the new work-hour restrictions really protect our trainees' quality of work and quality of life? Do they truly help protect our patients from receiving substandard care?

Frankly, I'd challenge either assumption.

On the one hand, I'd argue that there is an immediate downside to work-hour restrictions: our trainees no longer get an adequate exposure to training needed to become competent surgeons.

Have you ever heard the maxim that it takes 10,000 hours to successfully master something? Yes, 10,000 hours to become a qualified musician, painter, competitive athlete, or... *surgeon.*

The concept has been proven; it worked for the Beatles and for Bill Gates.[53]

Let's do the math (I love this part):

I'll look at the 551 surgical cases on my scorecard from 2014. For the sake of simplicity, I'll make the underlying assumption that an average case takes around 120 minutes 'skin-to-skin'. These 551 cases extrapolate to 1,102 hours of surgical experience per year, and to a total of 9 years to get me credentialed as a '10,000-hour' expert surgeon.

---

[52] Weinger MB, Ancoli-Israel S. Sleep deprivation and clinical performance. *JAMA* 2002; 287: 955-7.

[53] Gladwell M. *Outliers - The Story of Success.* New York, USA: Back Bay Books, 2008.

So you can tease me all you want about my lengthy residency training of 11 years. I'll counter that all those sleep-deprived, grueling years allowed me to get sufficient exposure to surgical cases.

10,000 hours.

That's how I learned 'to cut'.

Don't forget, we call our trainees "residents" because they were supposed to live 'in house' (i.e. at the hospital). This concept originated from the times of Osler and Halsted, the founders of the first medical residency program at Johns Hopkins in the late 19th century.

It's another no-brainer that the good ol' times of the "see one, do one, teach one" paradigm enabled residents to reach their 10,000-hour proficiency significantly faster than our modern-day trainees. Pragmatically speaking, we have simply traded our 'sleep-deprived' residents for 'case-deprived' residents.

Honestly, would you rather be operated on by an expert surgeon who's been on call the preceding night or by a 'semi-pro' who's well rested after an 8-hour beauty sleep?

Seriously, I'm asking you.

As the saying goes, during the first 10 years of training we learn *how* to cut, during the next 10 years in practice we learn *when* to cut, and during the last 10 years of our careers we learn *when not* to cut.

Dig this: 30 years to become a better surgeon!

And that's a stat from the pre-work-hour restriction age. Our modern-day residents may not even live long enough to reach the pinnacle of their learning curve.

And here's the true irony about this obsolete discussion: recent population-based studies suggest that sleep deprivation does not affect the quality of surgery or the risk of peri-operative complications. A

Canadian group from Ontario analyzed outcomes in 94,183 elective laparoscopic cholecystectomies performed by more than 300 community surgeons from 2004-2011.[54] The investigators analyzed 'at risk' cases performed by surgeons who operated between midnight and 7am the preceding night, and compared those with randomly matched procedures done by the same surgeons when they had not operated the night before.

And...?

There were *no differences* in the rate of intra-operative complications. And the risk of patients dying was in a similar range (around 0.1%), no matter whether their surgeon had rested the night before or not.

Seriously?!

Let me tell you a story to corroborate my personal conviction that surgeons can safely function after a sleepless night in our highly skilled and focused profession.

When I was as an attending trauma surgeon at the Benjamin Franklin University Hospital in Berlin, Germany, the concept of work-hour restrictions for residents was receiving increased nationwide attention. The year was 2003, and the ACGME had just rolled out the new work-hour restrictions for residents in the United States. In contrast, our residents in Germany were still taking 24-hour-call shifts and kept operating the next day. The widely publicized 'alcohol intoxication' analogy was causing an uproar in the German news media.

One day in the summer of 2003, the #1 ranked commercial TV station in Germany (RTL) approached our group with a request to follow a resident during a 24-hour-call shift. Their intent was to have a team of experts, including a neurologist and a nationally renowned sleep specialist, monitor the resident's level of sleepiness and quality of performance during a busy shift at a level 1 trauma center. Yohan Robinson, a 29-year-old junior resident in our team, volunteered for the

54 Vinden C, *et al.* Complications of daytime elective laparoscopic cholecystectomies performed by surgeons who operated the night before. *JAMA* 2013; 310: 1837-41.

task. The TV crew from RTL showed up to our ED the next day at 7am sharp. They 'hard-wired' Yohan with microphones and a dozen electrodes placed on his chest and onto the scalp over his head for continuous ECG and EEG monitoring (see the image below).

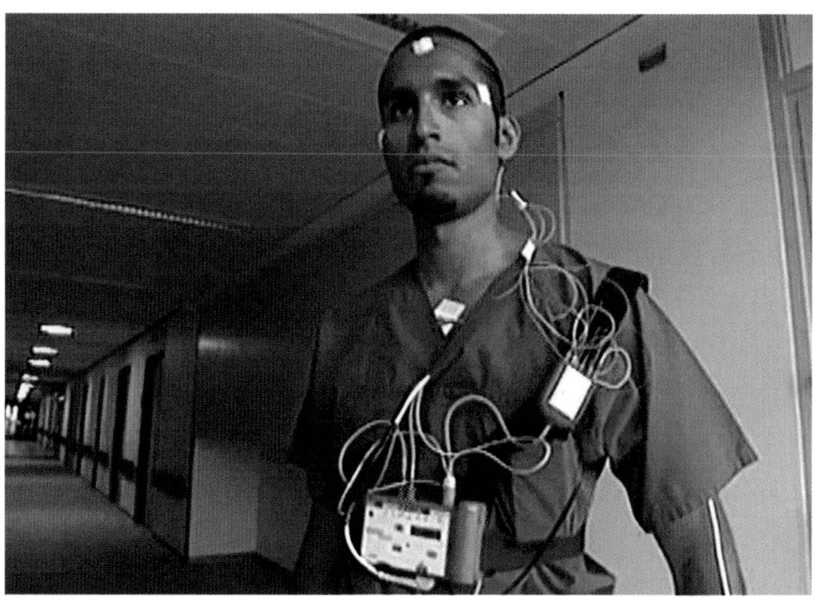

For the next 30 hours, the crew followed Yohan through the hospital. He didn't get 1 minute of sleep. During his shift, Yohan managed more than 70 patients with urgent and emergent conditions. The next day, as the crew unplugged him from the jungle of cables, Yohan stood tall and smiled. "This was a slam dunk — super fun! Thanks for the opportunity! Sorry guys, gotta go now — they're expecting me in the OR!"

The TV crew was astonished. The sleep specialist was speechless.

Yohan's heroic news coverage was broadcasted nationwide 2 weeks later.

The expert neurologist who interpreted the brain wave results for the TV audience was simply flabbergasted. "No change in EEG activity over 24 hours. Dr. Robinson's brain showed no signs of impaired level of operational capacity at any point in time. Looks like this particular resident is a complete exception from our understanding of the common effects of sleep deprivation. As a neurologist, I would clear him to start another consecutive 24-hour shift right away!"

Surprised?

I'm not. This seems to make perfect sense.

Think about it: all those studies that suggest that sleep deprivation is equivalent to alcohol intoxication actually looked at performance of monotonous routine tasks.[55] However, the simple extrapolation of these insights to the operating room is not really justified. Surgeons are distinct 'animals'. And the challenge of performing a surgical procedure is not equivalent to sitting in an office for a monotonous desk job, or driving a truck for 24 hours.

Surgeons don't tend to fall asleep in the operating room.

By now, most surgeons tend to agree that work-hour restrictions do not confer increased safety to our surgical patients and don't appear to make any sense from the perspective of quality of training for the next generation of surgeons.[56] This notion was confirmed in a recent systematic review of 27 studies published between 2011-2013 which revealed that the implementation of work-hour restrictions had:

- no impact on the quality of patient care;
- no impact on resident well-being; and
- an unfavorable impact on resident education.[57]

---

55 Veasey S, *et al.* Sleep loss and fatigue in residency training: a reappraisal. *JAMA* 2002; 288: 1116-24.

56 Businger AP, *et al.* Resident work-hour restrictions do not improve patient safety in surgery: a critical appraisal based on 7 years of experience in Switzerland. *Patient Safety in Surgery* 2012; 6: 17.

57 Bolster L, Rourke L. The effect of restricting residents' duty hours on patient safety, resident well-being, and resident education: an updated systematic review. *Journal of Graduate Medical Education* 2015; 7: 349-63.

Let me take this one step further: I'll argue that resident work-hour restrictions dramatically increase the risk of inflicting unintentional harm onto those it was originally designed to protect — our patients.

Our patients are the 'innocent bystanders' of another flawed system.

It all comes down to the imminent danger of increased *handovers* of care.

Consider the scenario in any teaching hospital these days: in the morning, the night float resident hands off the entire ward to the incoming daytime intern. This intern will then multi-task between numerous consults on inpatient wards and in the ED. The intern's only relevant goal will be to hand over the consult pager to the next intermittent shift house officer. And the job of baby-sitting the consult pager will be repeated again as the next incoming night float resident takes over.

All of these highly motivated young colleagues have one thing in common; they do not know the inpatients on the ward. Not only that; they have neither the training nor the time and luxury of providing *continuity of care* to their patients.

What I'm suggesting is that we're training a new generation of 'handover experts' who lack clinical expertise and personal accountability.

It's question-time again. Would you rather be cared for by an intern who is tired but knows you and your case in every meticulous detail, or by a rested intern who only knows your name from the handover list?

I know which option I'd choose.

Let's play this out further. We'll say that I am a postoperative patient admitted to the floor after a standard elective procedure, e.g. a laparoscopic cholecystectomy. You know that I'll be listed on the intern's handover sheet with the following hieroglyphs:

P.F.S. / 49-yom, POD#1 s/p lap chole, n.t.d.

Right, that's it.

The plan for the resident's engagement in my medical care is "n.t.d." — *nothing to do!*

Is it at all surprising that our trainees no longer learn empathy and compassion? They're playing an endless game of handovers, a game that can only be won by passing the consult pager like a 'hot potato' to the incoming resident who'll cover the next shift.

And considering all the multiple proven distractions during resident handovers,[58] we might as well call it a 'telephone game' with one certain loser: the patient.

So, tell me: are you in any way surprised that up to 440,000 patients die from medical errors in our hospitals every year? How many of those patients must have been listed as "n.t.d." on the intern's handover sheet in the dawn of their preventable death? We will never know, as dead patients are removed the very next morning from the updated handover list. It's a sobering thought. It's the stuff that keeps me up at night; the cause of my worst nightmares.

And yet, another dramatic example of a failed patient safety system.

In our ordinary lives it's easy to deal with 'system failure' — we simply reboot our PCs. Unfortunately, there is no 'reboot' button when the system fails to keep our patients safe.

[58] Anderson CE, *et al.* Distractions during resident handoffs: incidence, sources, and influence of handoff quality and effectiveness. *JAMA Surgery* 2015; 150: 396-401.

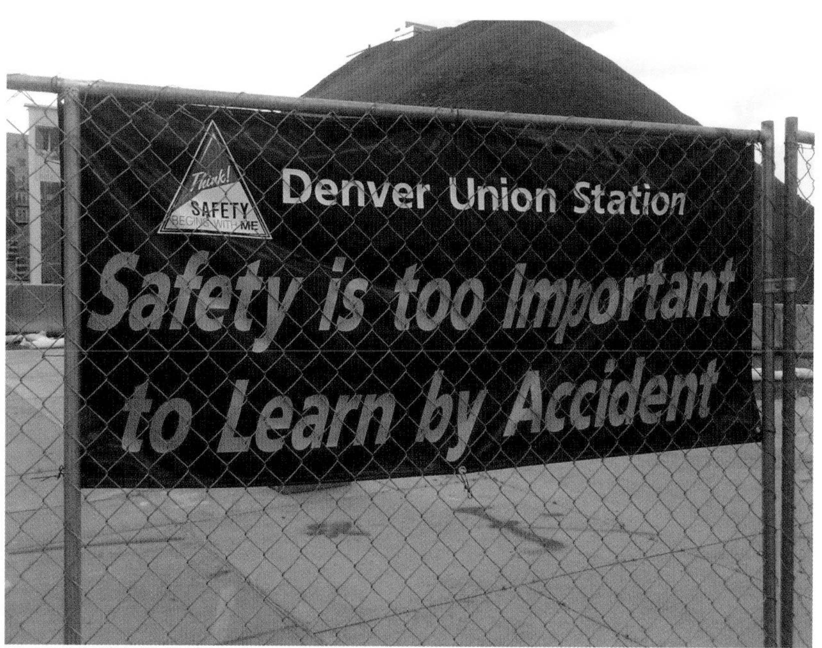
Think!
SAFETY
BEGINS WITH ME
Denver Union Station
Safety is too Important
to Learn by Accident

PART 5
The spiritual surgeon

Chapter 18 Your time is as valuable as my time

"Everyone thinks of changing the world but no one thinks of changing himself."

Leo Tolstoy (1828-1910)

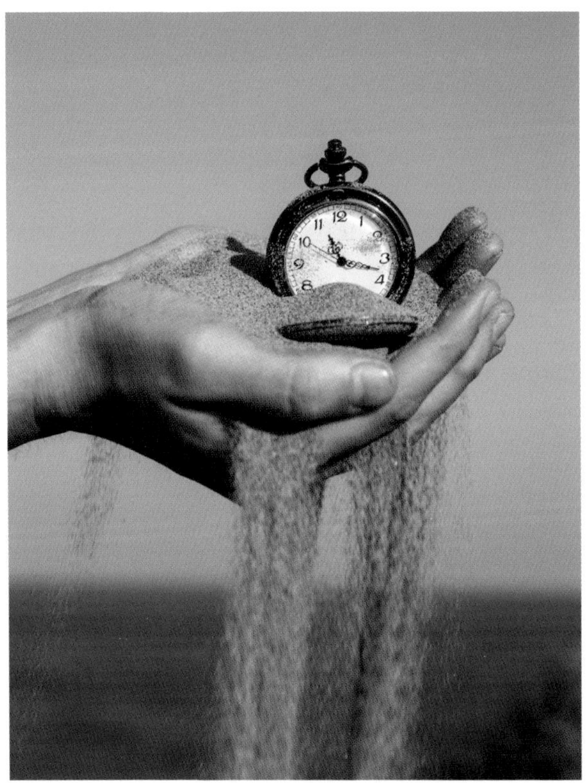

Surgeons are extremely privileged. There's no shame in saying it. But with privilege often comes a sense of entitlement.

Once we make it past medical school and residency training, it often feels as though the world is in our hands. The community typically looks up at us as they do to Marvel superheroes. Our staff and our patients continuously apologize to us for taking our 'important' time under the (erroneous) assumption that we are so extremely busy at all times.

This misconception has been cast in stone over generations.

Let me give you an example: on any given day at Denver Health, you might see me darting down the hall in green scrubs. Obviously I must be responding to an urgent OR call to save another life or limb. That's how important I am.

Right?

Well… What if I'm simply running down the hall to find the next available bathroom to accommodate a different sort of urgent matter?

Let's be honest: we can easily 'pull off' looking important 24/7 by simply wearing scrubs and projecting a demeanor of urgency wherever we go. Who would question our underlying motives?

It's true that we generally work our butts off for the sake of our patients. But how often is that not the case? How often do we modify our priorities purely for personal convenience?

After years of being told by our community how extremely important and 'busy' we are, this somewhat dangerous sense of entitlement can insinuate itself into our genome like a retrovirus. It's very easy to become the person you don't want to be.

One thing is certain: as surgeons, we have hundreds of daily tasks that keep us busy.

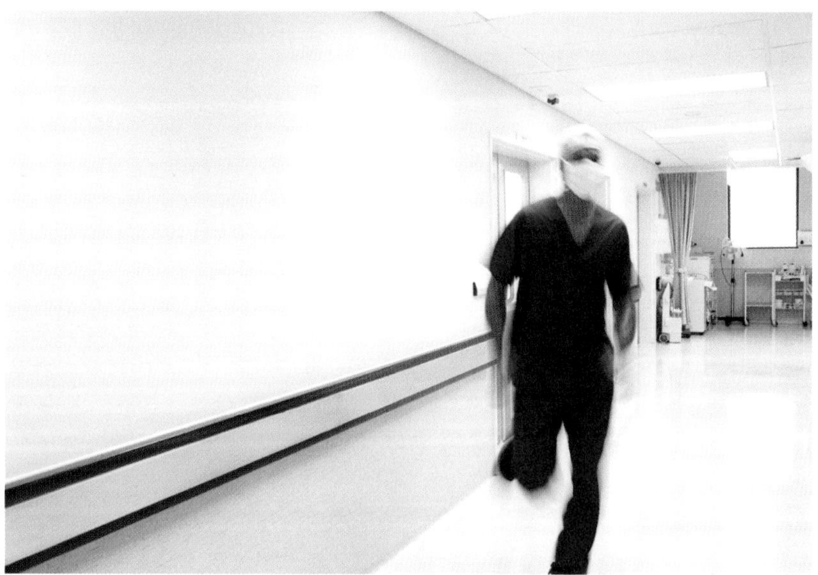

And guess what?

Most of them are not important at all.

Why is it reasonable to have a patient wait for us in the waiting room for a minute longer than we would be willing to wait ourselves? Have you ever seen a surgeon waiting patiently in front of an elevator or in line at a hotel's front desk? (The truth is, the term "patience" is not part of a surgeon's vocabulary.)

Yet, we impose unnecessary patience on to our patients and their families every day.

For many years over my surgical career, I learned a simple trick to hold myself accountable and to avoid falling into the 'trap of entitlement' in my respected profession. I live every day by the simple paradigm that: "your time is as valuable as my time."

What does this mean?

It means that we can change ourselves by purposefully changing our daily priorities.

We can start by dismissing the assumption that a surgeon's time is so dramatically more important than anyone else's. Instead of allowing a patient to wait in the office (so we can conveniently answer another email or deal with some other less important task), we can show respect for an individual patient's time, drop everything else immediately and go to see that waiting person.

I know, our patients make it too easy for us.

They typically forgive us the second we walk into the room for 'running late'. We don't even have to make up an excuse, owed to the general assumption that surgeons save lives on a daily basis. We are forgiven instantly.

In contrast, our front desk clerks and clinic staff 'in the trenches' get harassed endlessly for prolonged wait times. They take the heat for our tardiness.

What if we flip the roles around just for once?

What if the standard expectation was that surgeons should wait for their patients?

Let me illustrate this idea with a real example.

My friend Marc Pinto, whom I previously introduced, came to see me at Denver Health for a second opinion related to a complex injury he had sustained a week prior in a skiing accident.

I had never met Marc before. Yet when he arrived at Denver Health for his appointment, I was standing at the hospital entrance to personally greet him.

Sounds like a philosophical change of mindset; the surgeon waiting for the patient. But is this really a new revolutionary paradigm?

No. It's just the right thing to do.

We have to get rid of the hypocritical notion that it's OK to let patients wait based on the idea that they're designated *patients* because they're expected to be *patient*. Don't get me wrong, I have never been personally capable of eliminating wait times in my office on a particularly busy clinic day. However, I've stopped answering emails or taking care of other administrative duties when I know that patients are waiting for me. And I still apologize every day for running late, even though I'm not behind for my own convenience.

My simple rule of engagement is that if patients are waiting to see me, I will go to see them. Anytime and anywhere. The same is true for any family member waiting to meet with me to discuss the care of their loved ones.

Let me entertain you for a second with a true anecdote (the content is 100% accurate, whether you believe it or not). When I worked as a trauma surgeon in Berlin, Germany, I had a personal meeting with Professor Neuer,[59] a renowned surgeon and academician, to discuss an administrative issue.

As we were engaged in conversation in the Professor's office, his assistant interrupted us with an ad hoc request by an outside person to speak to him urgently. Professor Neuer was flabbergasted by the unexpected request and inquired who the person was.

The assistant told him that it was "the family of the patient you operated on this morning. They apparently haven't received any feedback and would like to talk to you to learn how the surgery went."

This message hit the fuel injector on Professor Neuer's ego-rocket.

He totally lost it right in front of my eyes. He jumped up and started yelling at his assistant. "A patient's family? Are you kidding me?" He shouted, "Do they know that I am a professor? Do they have the faintest

[59] Name changed to avoid any resemblance to actual individuals.

idea of how busy I am? Tell them that I have multiple important meetings and I clearly don't have time to talk to a patient's family."

Then he looked at me in a blank stare of disbelief.

"I just can't believe how people feel so entitled these days," he said as he rolled his eyes back in astonishment and mumbled: "Family members asking to speak to the professor... As if I had nothing else to do."

As Professor Neuer sat back down at his desk, his elbow accidentally tipped over a full cup of coffee. The liquid soaked most of the papers covering his desk.

This, of course, reignited his uncontrolled rage.

"God damn it!"

At this point, I was wishing that Scotty could 'beam me up' so I could vanish from my seat in the Professor's office. Sadly, there was no evident avenue of escape.

As I helped clean his desk, I saw that Neuer was chucking most of the coffee-soaked papers into the trashcan. He stratified the soaked papers by importance and mumbled his sorting strategy consistently as "not important... not important.... not important." I couldn't help but joke: "Professor, it's a good thing that none of these papers on your desk were apparently important at all."

That was an easy way out of his office.

Owing to such unpleasant experiences during my long path to become a better surgeon, I learned to trade the seductive (and unjustified) 'culture of entitlement' for an integral culture of respect for others.

Considering a patient's time as being as valuable as our own is simply a sign of respect. It is also a surrogate marker of *empathy*. There we are again, full circle back from our initial discussion in Part 1.

I just realized that I still owe you a practical tip on how to assess whether you're empathetic or not. Obviously, you can't simply fake empathy and hope to get away with it. The truth is, you can't fool your patients just as you can't fool your children. They both look up to you in respect, are dependent on you in many ways, and will therefore immediately 'call your bluff' if your apparent empathy is not genuine.

Patients, just like kids, can smell bullshit from miles away.

I can already hear you asking; if empathy can't be unequivocally defined and recognized, how the hell can we measure, quantify, and teach empathy to our trainees and students? It's too amorphous, too fuzzy.

Short answer: I don't think it is.

There are simple and pragmatic solutions.

While some people may instinctively argue that the extent of a person's dedication towards their pets and animals represents a reasonable surrogate marker for empathy towards all living creatures, I strongly challenge that. Just look at Adolf Hitler. He was extremely empathetic towards his beloved dog, Blondi. However, as the world would learn in horror and despair, he had no empathy or compassion for humankind.

So maybe empathy needs to be quantified differently.

It's been tried. Objective scoring systems like the Multifaceted Empathy Test or the Jefferson Scale of Physician Empathy exist. However, they're somewhat impractical and take time to learn and understand.

I actually have a much simpler and more pragmatic approach:

I call it the "Janitor Test".

Yes, janitor.

I believe that surgeons who aren't empathetic to every person they interact with on a daily basis won't be truly compassionate towards their patients either. They'll more likely portray a 'fake empathy' as part of an act delivered to their patients.

I have previously introduced my two janitor friends who work with me at Denver Health. For many years until present, David Frein has emptied the trash in my office and cleaned the hallways, and Mike McClain has cleared the trash and scrubbed the blood off the walls in our operating rooms. All told, I probably see the janitors who work in my building more often than I see my colleagues and family.

I assume the same is true for most of us.

Yet, unlike many of my surgeon colleagues, I really do know the janitors and greet them by their names every day. More than that, I know their hobbies, interests, family lives, and daily struggles. And they know mine. Both David and Mike work longer hours than I do. As I previously explained, both of them work several jobs to put a roof over their heads and food on their plates.

I've come to the conclusion that knowledge of the janitor's name is an excellent surrogate marker for determining whether a surgeon is empathetic towards others. Those who don't are conceivably perceived as arrogant or detached in the daily hum of a busy practice, with no time left to truly enjoy simple human interactions at a basic level.

You see where this is going, right?

Do you know your janitor's name?

I didn't think so.

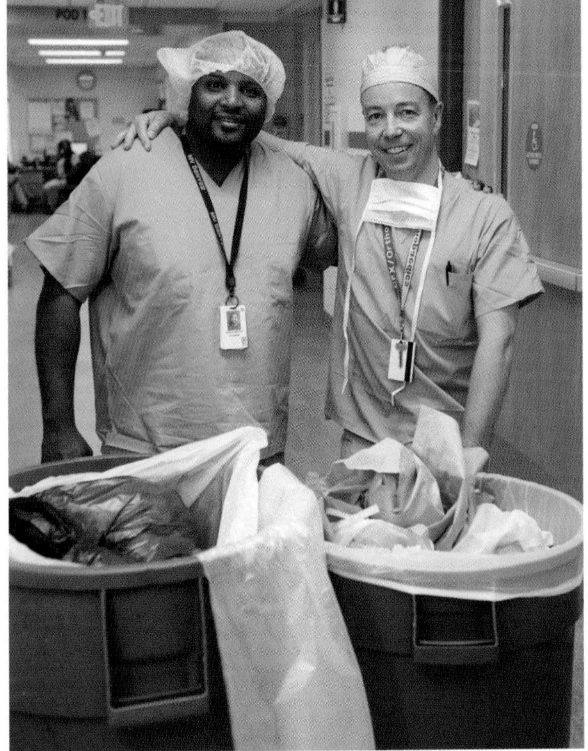

My janitor friend, Mike McClain, arguably the hardest working employee in our hospital.

So if you don't know your janitor's name and you're not empathetic, what are you? Well, people suffering from autism or paranoid schizophrenia are known to lack empathy.

At the risk of being provocative: should surgeons who are not emotionally engaged in the care of their patients be considered autistic or schizophrenic? (Fittingly enough, studies have shown higher scores for empathy in male psychiatrists than male surgeons.)

Look at it from a pragmatic perspective. A poor work/life balance and stressors in clinical practice directly contribute towards physician burnout and 'compassion fatigue', both of which appear to be significantly mitigated in physicians who have an inner spiritual balance driven by positive thinking.

This may sound like wishy-washy New Age drivel. I'm simply telling you that doctors who experience and live their lives as compassionate healers rather than purely technical surgeons are happier and last longer in their careers.

There is a famous Chinese proverb that supports the notion that it's never too late to change yourself:

"The best time to plant a tree was twenty years ago. The second best time is now!"

The next time you run into your janitor down the hallway, introduce yourself. Then, sit back, relax and observe your downstream transformation to becoming an empathetic surgeon.

Chapter 19 How to avoid burnout

"These are the duties of a physician: first, to heal his mind and to give help to himself, before giving it to anyone else."

Anonymous tombstone inscription in memory of an Athenian physician (2 AD)

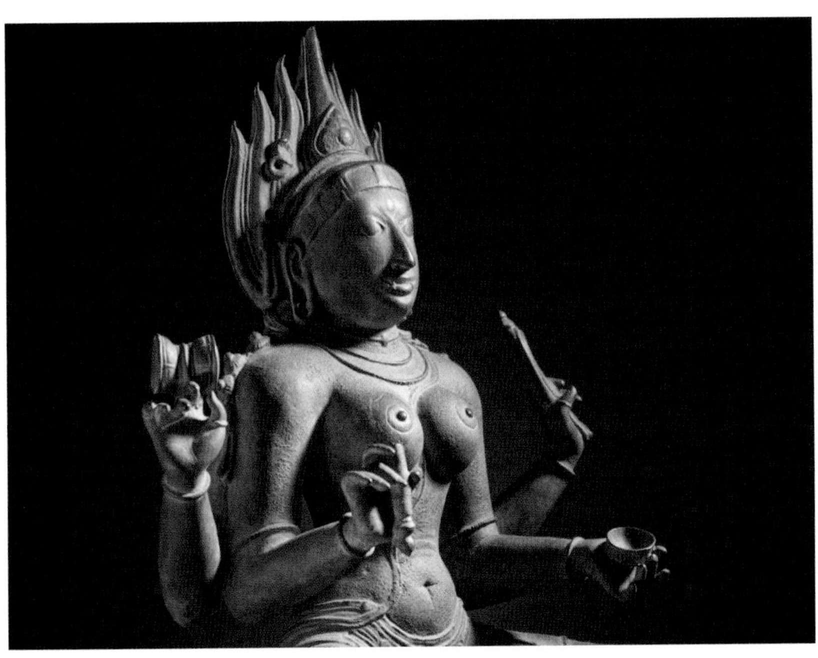

The practice of medicine is both extremely rewarding and highly challenging. Studies suggest about half of all physicians suffer from burnout, a poor quality of life, dissatisfaction with their work-life balance, and a high level of distress and fatigue.[60]

Believe it or not, about 20%-30% of all physicians have symptoms of depression.

There are, of course, downstream effects from the stress on physicians. Primarily, depression and fatigue often result in a lower quality of care delivered to patients and impaired competency and professionalism.

This sounds like a no-brainer. If we're stressed out and emotionally drained we won't have the energy and ability to carefully listen to our patients and incorporate their wishes and individual perspectives in their plan of care.

How can we heal others, if we can't heal ourselves?

I wish I was just making this stuff up but I'm not. Here's some of the evidence: a survey of 7,905 members of the American College of Surgeons revealed that the incidence of major medical errors is significantly increased in surgeons who report having a poor mental quality of life, burnout, and depression.[61]

Similar to other high-risk professions, surgeons generally don't deal with their own problems very well; they successfully ignore them.

Sound familiar? It did to me too.

In our profession we're known as being notoriously difficult patients regardless of our underlying illness. We even show up to work with a fever of 40°C — after all, that's what we're expected to do (frankly, I've never missed a single day of work for illness in 20 years).

---

[60] Shanafelt TD, *et al.* Burnout and satisfaction with work-life balance among U.S. physicians relative to the general U.S. population. *Archives of Internal Medicine* 2012; 172: 1377-85.

[61] Shanafelt TD, *et al.* Burnout and medical errors among American surgeons. *Annals of Surgery* 2010; 251: 995-1000.

In addition, we often take on more and more work on a daily basis and, unsurprisingly, feel invincible doing it. That is, until we break down under the accumulated weight of too many tasks and commitments.

Let me illustrate my point with a brief, insightful anecdote.

My good friend and esteemed colleague Dr. José Santiago is a retired 71-year-old psychiatrist from Spain. He's still active and engaged in spite of his relatively advanced age, flying across the United States as a hospital consultant and exercising on his road bike several days a week. Needless to say, José is in admirable physical and mental shape.

During a recent visit to Denver, José came to see me in my office for a sore knee he'd developed following a brutal bike trek. After the consultation, we sat and chatted about work and life for a while. José told me an intriguing story based on his decades in practice. As a psychiatrist, he'd treated many surgeons who sought counseling for a variety of mental conditions related to distress, depression, fatigue, and burnout. As he started his anecdote, José looked at me, smiled, and pointed to the cup of steaming black coffee I'd just poured a minute prior.

"That's exactly what I did when I greeted a surgeon as my new patient on the first visit," he said. "I'd pour a cup of coffee and hold it in my hand during the entire consultation."

I gave José a confused look. I didn't get where he was going with this.

"After the first session, I would generally ask the surgeon what he thought I was holding in my hand." José smiled. "And I would invariably get the same answer, that the cup of coffee is *half full*. Ha! You surgeons are smart people and can't be fooled easily with a standard trick question on positive thinking. But that's not where I was going with my question."

I admit that I was a bit embarrassed as I was about to give the intuitive "half-full" answer myself. Good thing I hadn't missed my opportunity to shut up and listen.

"My next question to the surgeon would be to ask him to guess the weight of this half cup of coffee. Around 6 ounces? Sounds about right?"

I nodded.

"Well, then, how long do you think I could possibly hold this 6-ounce cup of coffee in my hand? Obviously, I had been holding it with ease for about an hour during our preceding conversation. What's your estimate? Another hour? For the rest of the day? For a full week? That's absolutely impossible! Even if I was a world-champion body builder, I would not be able to hold a 6-ounce cup of coffee that long, and certainly not for an entire career."

It suddenly dawned on me: José was alluding to our mindset, our deep-seated belief that as surgeons we can deal with any problem any time, no matter how urgent and important. The fact is: surgeons will never admit to being over-burdened with tasks; instead, we apply the standard Wild West *modus operandi*, requesting our opponents to just "bring it on!"

Yeah, that's definitely familiar.

But eventually all the minor assignments and seemingly small tasks that we accept every day without hesitation catch up with us. Like the constant weight of a half-full cup of coffee, these accumulations are easy to carry day-by-day, and absolutely impossible to carry for a lifetime! Given enough time, even we eventually drop the 6-ounce cup on the floor... and when that happens it's generally too late.

No use trying to save spilled coffee.

I got José's message loud and clear.

As I escorted him to the door, he turned around and gave me a stern look. "We have to start fixing small things in our lives, day-by-day. Nobody changes overnight!" As José turned around and left my office, I quickly emptied my half cup of coffee in one single sip, intent on abolishing the symbolic cause of my looming burnout.

I've personally witnessed many experienced surgeons hit a breaking point after many successful years in practice. The ones I knew started hating themselves and developed grudges against their practice, their coworkers, and their patients. They traded their positive spirit as *healers* for a negative and miserable existence as *haters*.

Let me tell you a horrifying story about the risk of allowing decision-makers in high-risk industries to become distressed and depressed:

On March 24, 2015, the commercial passenger flight Germanwings 9525 was deliberately steered into the French Alps by a suicidal co-pilot who suffered from chronic depression and had been previously declared "unfit to work" by his psychiatrist.

He killed all 150 people on board.

He was unfit to work.

It's a frightening diagnosis. Would you ever want to be under the knife of a surgeon who was declared mentally unfit to work? I'm not going to suggest that depressed surgeons are at risk of massacring their patients, but I am saying that burned-out surgeons are a danger to their patients.

Burnout is ugly. I still remember my first exposure to it.

I was a 26-year-old medical student on my first elective clinical rotation in internal medicine at a regional hospital on the picturesque shore of Lake Zurich. My direct supervisor, Veronica,[62] was a charming resident in her early 30s, just a couple years away from finishing her training with the goal of being board-certified as an internist.

Veronica appeared infinitely dedicated to the care of her patients. She was genuinely empathetic, not only to her colleagues and peers, but also to each and every patient under her watch. Even though I was a 'know-nothing rookie', within a few weeks of working with Veronica, I noticed hints of fatigue and exhaustion in her behavior. I suspected that the demanding day-to-day job in the trenches might have started taking its toll,

62 Name changed to avoid any resemblance to actual individuals.

which is ironic, as I was completely overwhelmed with my own assignments on my elective rotation at the time. Thrown into a busy hospital with unclear expectations and an overwhelming number of clinical assignments, I had no clue what I was doing.

Seriously.

I remember spending 2 hours in an exam room with my first internal medicine patient to complete an admission H&P. At the end of the exam, my elderly patient told me that in his 75 years he'd never undergone such a detailed clinical exam. He was delighted.

Ha!

What I took as a compliment at the time was clearly nothing more than a shining example of my inexperience and ineffectiveness in succinctly completing my job.

Four weeks into my rotation and after an exhausting weekend on call, I left the hospital to get a few hours of sleep prior to my next shift. As I stepped out through the impressive neoclassical stairwell of the hospital's main entrance, I found Veronica sitting on the stairs with her head in her lap, sobbing.

Clearly, something was wrong.

I was embarrassed and had no idea how to respond.

Today, I would have just walked up to her, given her a warm hug, and reassured her that she would be fine. She likely just needed some rest. Back then, however, I stood awkwardly on the stairwell, wondering if I should blurt out some meaningless question like "Everything OK?"

It was very obvious that nothing was close to being "OK".

Like a coward, I snuck over to the railway station and took the local train back to my student home in Zurich. I just wanted to forget what I'd seen.

I was too overwhelmed with the situation and embarrassed about my own behavior. When I arrived back at the hospital around 6pm the same night, Veronica was "MIA".

She didn't return to work the next day either.

Forty-eight hours later, the Department Head called an impromptu team huddle and told us that Veronica had unexpectedly decided to quit the training program.

I was stunned.

I was still 2 years away from the preventable death of my ICU patient in my first shift as a doctor. Still fresh, still convinced I could take on the world. It was shocking to me that Veronica's medical career, her life's mission as a healer, had been abruptly extinguished in the blazing flames of *physician burnout* on a warm summer day under the gorgeous blue skies covering Lake Zurich...

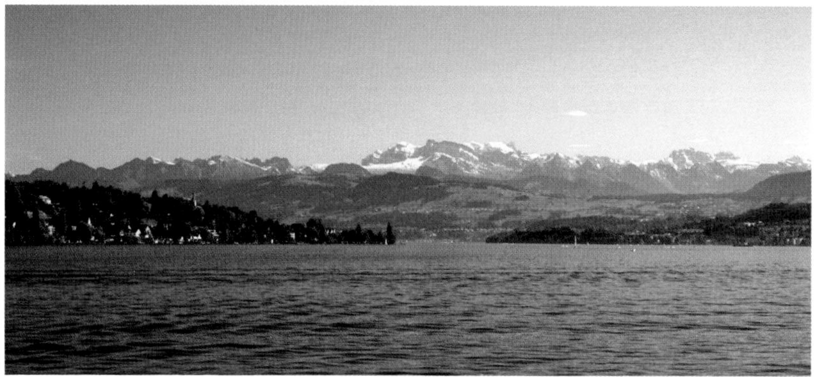

What struck me most about Veronica's experience was the fact that even young residents with only a few years of completing their training are at risk of burnout. All my life I had erroneously assumed that this fate was reserved for older guys like me, guys beyond the peak of their careers who are looking forward to early retirement.

I recently took a minute to investigate this problem more scientifically.

Entering the terms "surgeon burnout" and "resident burnout" into my PubMed search engine, articles about residents trumped articles on surgeons' burnout by 189 to 149 in terms of retrieved publications. These results were pale compared to my search for "medical student burnout". This query came back with 278 publications on PubMed.

If you look at the underlying root cause of burnout among medical professionals early in their careers, it's a high level of emotional pressure combined with the challenge of sustaining a meaningful work-life balance.[63]

Same stuff. All over again.

In a somewhat perverse way, it makes sense that the medical students who prevail (those successfully avoiding burnout) tend to be the same students who lose their empathy in the third year of medical school (as previously discussed: "The devil is in the third year"). And for surgeons, I believe the risk of burnout is easily doubled, compared to non-interventional specialists.

Not only are we expected to perform at the highest level of impeccable quality at all times, but we're inundated with ever-changing regulations. Currently we have to manage the integration of electronic health records (EHR) in clinical practice, fulfill the requirements for coherent documentation, regulatory compliance, oversight and billing. Provocatively speaking, we have been thrown into a *Hunger Games* equivalent fight for survival in a dramatically growing and financially competitive health care market driven by benchmarks that are largely outside a surgeon's control. That's not even touching on the increasing threat from the medicolegal industry.

With the patient's best interest in mind, we balance on a daily basis 'when to cut' against the option of observation and non-operative management. Clearly, we remain vulnerable to a medicolegal claim from

[63] Dyrbye LN, *et al.* Burnout among U.S. medical students, residents, and early career physicians relative to the general U.S. population. *Academic Medicine* 2014; 89: 443-51.

either decision. Waiting and observing instead of operating immediately bears the risk of a claim for delayed or inaccurate diagnosis and tardy initiation of treatment. On the other hand, patients can be exposed to serious and potentially preventable surgical complications when taken to the operating room preemptively.

In many years of practice, I've seen many esteemed colleagues at the edge of burnout due to a disconnect between their ability to provide high-quality care to their patients and the need to mitigate their own legal risk of being sued for perceived negligent care.

I vividly remember the terrifying moment when I was presented with my own first notice of a legal claim. I'd just taken my surgical board exams a year prior and was a young and enthusiastic attending trauma surgeon intending to heal all my patients in my role as a 'noble knight'. One of our ED nurses, Antje,[64] had been bugging me for a while about scoping her knee for chronic pain. I'd seen her in my office, examined her knee and documented the findings. I found no relevant indication that would justify a surgical procedure. She kept bothering me every time I ran into her. It took several months of persistent complaining but Antje finally persuaded me to proceed with a diagnostic knee arthroscopy.

What a mistake!

The procedure was straightforward and, if anything, just confirmed my initial impression that her knee was bothering her due to some chronic 'wear and tear'. When I disclosed these intra-operative findings, Antje inexplicably became upset. She avoided any further interaction with me at work, and within a couple of months, filed a notice of claim through our risk management department. She claimed that I'd delayed the surgical procedure and therefore contributed to a prolonged period of unnecessary suffering.

Gulp.

Only later did I realize that Antje had been driven by a hidden agenda. She wanted to retire early and use a 'debilitating medical condition' as her

[64] Name changed to avoid any resemblance to actual individuals.

way out. When my intra-operative findings failed to match what she wanted to hear, she switched gears and went for financial gain. While the surgical procedure had gone well and there had been no medical error or surgical complication, the end result was still an unhappy patient. It was a rookie mistake on my part; a clear lapse in judgment.

The notice of claim really threw me out of bounds.

I couldn't sleep for weeks. I assumed my career was already over. And if it wasn't, I dreaded the thought that I would lose all respect at the hospital where I worked. Antje was a senior nurse. She was respected and well liked by her peers. I just knew she'd continue defaming my clinical skills and reputation among our staff. Even worse, my ego was bruised. I was under the impression that I had failed to heal a patient and that the care I provided had actually not been beneficial, but rather the opposite.

I remember that I was my own worst critic during the painful and lengthy process that followed. At the time, only two things kept me from spinning entirely out of control.

First was the consoling mentorship of one of my senior partners in whom I had confided. He unequivocally helped me keep my mental sanity through incredibly tough times by assuring that this "happens to the best of us" and appealing to "never give up".

Second was my scrutiny and diligence in written documentation. I had documented everything in Antje's chart, including her preceding clinic encounters and detailed notes about the formal shared decision-making process for surgery. It was ultimately this diligence that would end up clearing my name. Our risk management experts attested that my documentation was impeccable and clarified that there had been no deviation from the standard of care. The claim was eventually dropped by the plaintiff.

Imagine what would have happened to my career if I had consulted Antje as a 'curbside' undocumented favor to a respected coworker? By sheer luck, the claim dissolved in air and I only suffered a couple of months of sleepless nights with a bottle of prescription medication from my primary care physician to control my first (and so far only) episode of severe anxiety.

This painful episode reflects three important concepts in terms of dealing with medicolegal issues that can lead to burnout:

- Most claims and lawsuits are not based on medical errors (as in my personal story above). Reciprocally, most medical errors or surgical complications never end up in a claim or lawsuit.
- Only written documentation keeps us out of trouble. From a judge's perspective, anything that isn't documented in writing, never happened.
- My anecdotal story emphasizes the classic analogy of the 'two victims' theory: the *patient* who suffered (real or perceived) harm, and the *surgeon* whose spiritual life and mental balance are suddenly and dramatically derailed (as previously portrayed by Dr. Jimmy Reed's anecdotal example).[65]

Following on from these thoughts, I recently screened the published literature on the physician specialties most vulnerable to patient lawsuits. It didn't take me long to see that I hadn't been a lone ranger exposed to the horrific experience of a notice of claim.

A wide-ranging study published in 2011 analyzed a professional liability insurance database of 40,916 physicians and 233,738 covered physician-years.[66] During a 15-year study period, 7.4% of all physicians had been exposed to a malpractice claim. The 'top-5' specialties at risk were exclusively surgical disciplines, with neurosurgeons and cardiothoracic surgeons at highest risk for a claim (around 19%!), followed by general surgeons, orthopaedic surgeons, and plastic surgeons.

This means that almost one in five surgeons are sued over a period of 15 years. To put it another way, if you practice long enough, you will

---

65 Pinto A, *et al.* Acute traumatic stress among surgeons after major surgical complications. *American Journal of Surgery* 2014; 208: 642-7.

66 Jena AB, *et al.* Malpractice risk according to physician specialty. *New England Journal of Medicine* 2011; 365: 629-36.

receive a notice of claim in the mail. No matter how indestructible you think you are, getting such a letter can initiate or propagate a downward spiral of mental distress that may easily lead to burnout and subsequent detrimental sequelae.

So what then is the most effective remedy to prevent or mitigate this potentially detrimental downward spiral?

The peer-reviewed literature offers a variety of approaches on spiritual healing, though none appear practically feasible for a busy surgeon 'in the trenches'. We certainly have the opportunity of joining a Balint group or to attend Schwartz Center rounds for caregivers' mental support. These are the important existing structures designed to help us navigate the tricky waters of burnout.

There is no way, however, that I could see myself (or any of my respected surgical colleagues, for that matter) sitting in a group of peers and analyzing our daily stressors and mental challenges. How about the recommendation of listening to music during daily yoga and meditation sessions in a so-called "guilt-free timeout" between patient encounters? Please understand, I don't mean to ridicule such practices. If they work for some people, that's fantastic. I don't think they work for *busy surgeons.*

You might take a look in a bookstore for a guide on spiritual health but that's not a simple task either. Which book should you buy? There are literally tens of thousands of books dedicated to the topic. Take a minute and search your online book store; Amazon alone will retrieve more than 35,000 hits on "spiritual health".

Of all these books, I identified a selected few that I found helpful on my path to become a better surgeon and spiritual physician. These include Robin S. Sharma's classic fable *The Monk Who Sold His Ferrari* (1997), Captain Dan Willis' *Bulletproof Spirit* (2014), and my Denver Health friend and colleague Abraham Nussbaum's outstanding essay, *The Finest Traditions of My Calling* (2016).

So what have I found effective in my own life?

How do I keep burnout at bay?

I still enjoy getting up early every day and dedicating long working hours to a mix of clinical care, administrative duties, and research projects. I take regular 24-hour call shifts, one weekday a week, and a three-day weekend every month. And I have fun doing it.

People who work with me will see me smile all day long.

What's the secret of my success?

For the sake of simplicity, I'll stratify my own personal recipe against burnout into *seven* distinct 'ingredients'.

1. Discipline and rituals

> "The way of life I preach is a habit to be acquired gradually by long and steady repetition. It is the practice of living for the day only. Do the day's work well and don't worry about tomorrow."
>
> **Sir William Osler (1849-1919)**

As I mentioned previously in the book, Dr. Osler figured it all out more than a 100 years ago. Anything that I will ever have to say (or write; including the core content of this book), Osler already knew. If we follow his guiding principles, we will be productive, effective, and happy. (In this regard, the best biography I've read about Osler's legacy is by Charles S. Bryan; it's truly a 'must read' for any medical student and physician in training and practice.)[67]

One of Osler's most pragmatic imperatives, in my opinion, is reflected by the opening quote above. Work hard every day, do your work well, and never worry about the future. Worrying about tomorrow doesn't accomplish anything. Similarly, there is no dwelling on past occurrences. Anxiety about the future and regret about the past only distract us from our focus on the job we have to do today.

---

[67] Bryan CS. *Osler - Inspirations from a Great Physician.* Oxford, UK: Oxford University Press, 1997.

Hector's got it down. He's my little Chihuahua dog. And though he weighs less than 5 pounds, he's a more spiritual individual than I can ever be. I'm not kidding. Hector, like all dogs, lives in the present 100% of the time. He never worries about the future and has no regrets about the past. The guy is insanely happy and appears infinitely fulfilled every minute of the day.

In all seriousness, everything we do comes down to the moment, the 'now'. Discipline and rituals allow us to get the job done every day, consistently and effectively. We can't succeed with important goals if we don't put positive pressure on ourselves. And pressure is not always a bad thing; it drives discipline and rituals. This inspires us to overcome insurmountable barriers and achieve unimaginable goals. This is how we create our legacy. And ultimately, our legacy is all we have. It's our meaning of life.

As valuable as they are, rituals only really catch on if you practice them without exception for at least 30 consecutive days.[68]

This is a proven rule. Once you make the 30-day mark, you own the ritual. No bullshit. This is why New Year's resolutions never catch on — most people don't follow through until February 1. It's so easy and tempting to slip back into our comfortable old habits. That's where discipline comes into play.

So what sort of rituals am I talking about? Simple ones. Rituals that will guide your day and allow you to accomplish each day's work without wasting your time:

- Get up early and go to bed at the same time every day.
- Read before you fall asleep. The last thoughts of your day will accompany you through the night until the next morning. (This is also why you shouldn't fall asleep watching TV.)
- Spend 30 minutes a day reading 'real' books, not just the daily medical literature, magazines and newspapers. As Osler stated:

---

[68] Sharma RS. *The Monk Who Sold His Ferrari.* New York, USA: HarperOne, 1997.

"Start at once a bed-side library and spend the last half hour of the day in communion with the saints of humanity."

- Dedicate 30 minutes a day listening to music. Actively. I have never met a depressed or distressed person who actively listens to music. It's spiritual health for your soul.
- Dedicate 30 minutes a day to writing — not emails or research papers, but your own thoughts, plans for the day, and your long-term vision of what you want your legacy to be. (For this purpose, my daily companions are a quality fountain pen and a notebook.)
- Spend 30 minutes briefing and debriefing your day (15 minutes each). The briefing session will define your tentative plan and expectations for the coming day and give you the positive energy needed. The debriefing will allow you to look back at what you truly accomplished and what you've learned. Doing this step-by-step, day-by-day, allows you to modify your course as needed, in case things don't go as planned (as happens invariably in a surgeon's hectic and unpredictable practice).

Sounds too demanding and too complicated?

Well, here's another catch: all rituals have to be accomplished in isolation without any distraction or interruption. For example, my own briefing/debriefing rituals work best under the shower, where I can think unbothered, and envision the water to wash away any negative energy. That's why I take the luxury of taking two showers per day (I apologize if this is too much information for the reader!). Hydrophobic people can accomplish the same ritual in a dark corner of the house or apartment, as exemplified by the daily habits of one of my heroes, Benjamin Franklin.

I know what's coming next. You want me to tell you where exactly to find the additional 2 hours to accomplish all these rituals. Fair enough.

Well, here are two pragmatic options:

For starters, stop wasting hours dedicating your attention to issues of little importance. How about sacrificing a part of the 4.9 hours of TV watching we average every day? And if you're not willing to give up the TV? Well, then, get up earlier! This is where rituals meet discipline. Remember, early awakening is the first ritual on my list. It's up to you to decide if 'early' means 4am (as do some of my most productive friends; I just don't have the discipline), 5am (my own wake-up time), or 6am (probably shouldn't be much later than that).

There is an ancient Chinese proverb that hits the spot about this ritual:

> "No one who rises before dawn 360 days a year fails to make his family rich."

Keep in mind that sleep is really nothing more than a habit. And habits can be whipped into shape with discipline. You will always feel uncomfortable when you initiate a new ritual. That's normal. But when it hits the 30-day mark, it'll be intrinsic.

And if you're tempted to abandon a ritual, keep in mind the distinction between barriers and excuses. *Barriers* are challenges (and at the same time opportunities) to incentivize us to pursue and achieve higher goals. In contrast, *excuses* incentivize the opposite, namely to give in to discipline for the sake of pure convenience (or laziness). The two can appear identical to the untrained eye. It's up to you to distinguish between a cheap excuse versus a real opportunity disguised as a barrier.

Clearly, life is too short to miss out on opportunities!

2. Positive thinking

> "When you are enthusiastic about what you do, you feel this positive energy. It's very simple."
>
> **Paolo Coelho (*1947)**

Positive thinking is the main driver of all valuable goals in life.

Dig this: it's as easy to think positively as it is to think negatively. But there is a decisive difference that goes beyond ease: positive energy always eradicates negative energy.

Consider that the only thing we can control in our lives as human beings is that we have absolute control over our own minds. By controlling our minds, we control our thoughts. If you Google how many thoughts humans have you'll find a consensus of around 50,000 thoughts per day. And guess what? More than 90% of these thoughts are either negative, repetitive, or irrelevant. Most of our thoughts deal with stuff we can't change like issues from the past and worries about the future. By choosing to live and act in the present we can clear our minds and focus on positivity.

A couple of weeks ago I was on call over a long holiday weekend. During a fourth night in the operating room crammed with long turnover times between cases and little sleep, I ran into my janitor friend Mike McClain. It was 2am.

"What's up Doc? Why are you here during the holidays?"

Instead of complaining about my misfortune, I smiled at him and said: "I love working nights because I get to interact with nice people like you!"

We are what we think and we become what we think about.

The Roman Emperor and stoic philosopher, Marcus Aurelius, was quoted as saying that we can't always control the events around us, but we can control how we react to them. This couldn't be more applicable to the life of a 21st century surgeon. Our profession makes us extremely vulnerable to negative energy. It can stick to our backs like glue. And there is only one way to eradicate negative energy: by *positive thinking*.

The way you can do this is essentially by prioritizing your daily allocation of 5,000 meaningful thoughts over the 45,000 other, irrelevant thoughts. It takes a conscious effort aimed at protecting your positive spirit to stop from being diluted or contaminated by all the basic stuff that keep your mind busy throughout the day.

I'm not going to pretend it's easy. It clearly isn't.

It's a tough exercise that requires daily practice and conscious commitment and dedication. If you're angry at your peers, your administrators, or even at your patients, just step aside and look in the mirror: what you think about others says more about yourself than about the others. Thus, you need to change your thoughts.

As discussed about rituals, we must block out 30 minutes per day for clearing and prioritizing our thoughts. The success of this venture relies on the next prerequisite for a healthy spirit: awareness.

3. Awareness

> "The ultimate value of life depends upon awareness rather than upon mere survival."
>
> **Aristotle (384 BC-322 BC)**

Have you ever been really sick?

So sick that all the things you planned to do just vanished under the exclusive desire to be healthy again? Do you remember what the first day after your recovery felt like? When you stepped outside and took a deep breath, enjoyed the sunlight on your face, and paid attention to stuff you'd never consider on a 'regular' busy work day; like observing the clouds in the sky, listening to birds chirping from the trees, and enjoying the sight of children laughing and random people chatting?

Do you remember how unconditionally happy you were in that instant?

It must have been the living in the moment, without distraction, judgment or worry. Well, if you have ever been through this scenario, then you probably had the opportunity to experience *full awareness*. The problem is that we hardly dedicate any time and energy to awareness in our hectic lives as surgeons. You probably don't even remember how fast that feeling evaporated after the next overwhelmingly busy day with meetings and administrative and clinical duties. The half-life of awareness is so extremely short, that once you think about it, it's already gone.

We take all the fundamental things in life for granted. The 'delta' change in our well-being after we recover from illness makes all the difference. However, you don't have to wait to catch the flu to achieve this goal; as for positive thoughts, you can practice and condition awareness. This is a pure mental trait. As you build your muscles with regular exercise, you can train yourself through the different stages of awareness:

- *Stage 1* reflects a rudimentary and constricted level of awareness. This is when we struggle with daily issues and (over)react to every problem with anxiety and defensiveness.
- *Stage 2* consists of a broadening awareness, when we see beyond the problem in front of us and come up with positive and meaningful solutions.
- *Stage 3* means that we made it; we achieve pure awareness when there are no problems, no struggles, and no fear; all negative thoughts and worries have been exchanged for unconditional love for the life we live in.

I have a daily awareness ritual that I practice after my morning briefing. I step outside into the fresh morning air, look up to the sky, and fill my lungs with three deep breaths of fresh air. Then, I enjoy my drive to work with dedicated awareness to all my surroundings. No angry administrator, disgruntled coworker, annoying meeting, or change in the weather can interfere with my positive experience for the rest of the day.

Try it out. It works!

4. Empathy, generosity, and gratitude

> "Be strong, be kind, be generous, be understanding, and let people know how grateful you are."
>
> **George H.W. Bush (*1924)**

I'm not going to perseverate here about the crucial role of empathy in becoming a better surgeon; we've already gone over it in depth in the first part of the book.

Let's rather talk about empathy in the context of avoiding burnout.

Consider how your level of empathy positively affects your own spiritual well-being. If you are kind and empathetic to other people, the positive energy you donate to others will be reflected back at you. The same is true with generosity — if you are generous (a surrogate marker of your empathy), you will feel great simply based on the fact that you want others to be happy and to do well.

When was the last time you gave money to a homeless beggar on the street?

Do you remember the joy and gratitude in that person's eyes?

And do you remember how good you felt about yourself afterwards, with the person's sincere gratitude echoing in your mind ("Thank you, sir… God bless you, sir… Have a wonderful day, sir!"). If you're looking for the perfect antidote to burnout, you've found a remedy.

Let's hear it from the master Dr. Osler himself: "We can best oppose any tendency of melancholy by an active life of unselfish devotion to others."

Last but not least, don't underestimate the power of gratitude.

Gratitude heals the soul and sustains our purpose of life. We have so many things to be grateful for. There is not a single interaction or discussion that I have with others where I don't end with a brief "Thank you!"

And since I have dozens of meetings and discussions every day, I never miss an opportunity to say thank you. As a matter of fact, nobody ever leaves my office without getting a formal "Thank you!" on the way out.

And I have not regretted it once.

5. Decisiveness and perseverance

> "Permanence, perseverance, and persistence in spite of all obstacles, discouragements, and impossibilities: it is this that in all things distinguishes the strong soul from the weak."
>
> **Thomas Carlyle (1795-1881)**

As surgeons, we learn early in our careers to be decisive.

We make quick decisions with confidence.

It takes a certain breed of people to have the decisiveness and bravado to 'cut another human open' in the face of uncertainty. It's who we are and it's what distinguishes us from non-surgical disciplines in the medical profession.

This characteristic protects us from the dangers of indecision; dangers associated with uncertainty and anxiety. The apparent downside of being overly decisive is the risk of poor judgment and erroneous decision-making. Both can potentially harm our patients. This dichotomy remains a surgeon's ultimate 'moment of truth' as we attempt to quantify and mitigate risk and uncertainty (see Part 2 of the book).

Likewise, perseverance is reflected in our eternal determination to do the right thing for our patients and to "never surrender" (Churchill) in the face of recurring obstacles and barriers. Perseverance always pays off. And this is most suitably reflected in a classic quote by John Rockefeller:

> "I do not think that there is any other quality as essential to success of any kind as the quality of perseverance. It overcomes almost everything, even nature."

6. Time management

> "I have two kinds of problems: the urgent and the important. The urgent are never important and the important are never urgent."
>
> **Dwight D. Eisenhower (1890-1969)**

Time is the most precious resource in life.

No human being can save time.

People say that "time is money" but that's a misconception because you can't deposit time into a savings account and use it later. In our busy lives as surgeons, we tend to forget that time is a non-renewable resource. Everyone has 24 hours per day at their disposal.

What distinguishes people who achieve high goals is that they take better advantage of their available time compared to the average population. Peter Turla, the President of the National Management Institute, corroborated this notion in a fitting quote: "Managing your time without setting priorities is like shooting randomly and calling whatever you hit the target."

If you want to use your time effectively, the principles that guide your life will also drive your goals; in turn, your goals will determine your priorities; and your priorities will help you decide what you do with your day.

Remember, your legacy is nothing more than the sum of what you achieved on individual days.

President Eisenhower provided a simple scheme for prioritization of daily tasks based on their importance and urgency. Using the Eisenhower Decision Matrix (see the figure below), you can easily stratify your tasks based on whether they are urgent (or not) and important (or not).

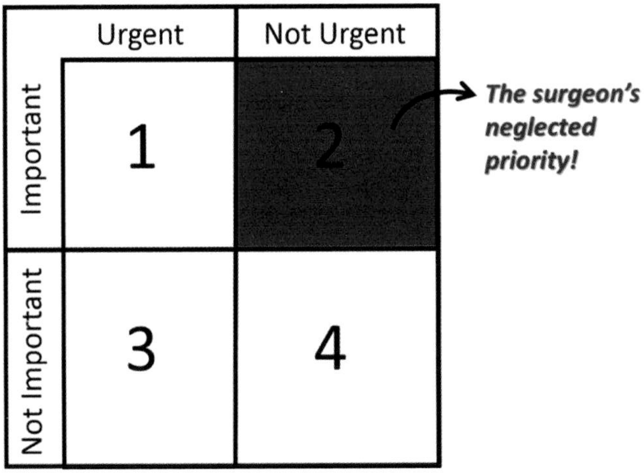

	Urgent	Not Urgent
Important	1	2
Not Important	3	4

The surgeon's neglected priority!

The "Eisenhower Principle" for prioritization of daily tasks.

Of the four resulting options, two are no-brainers: Box 1 (the *'to do'* box) summarizes all tasks that are urgent and important, such as going to the operating room when there is a patient on the table or to the outpatient clinic when a patient is waiting. There is no alternative; you just have to do it.

Similarly, box 4 (the *'to eliminate'* box) is easy to handle: these are the daily time fillers such as surfing the internet, wasting time on social media, or watching entertainment shows on TV (I'm hopefully not offending any readers!). These tasks should be simply eliminated if we are truly determined to manage our time well.

I'll give you a quick and practicable example of how I diminished the quantity of my daily box 4 tasks: I stopped reading emails that I'm only copied on. It's easy: you just have to think outside of your inbox. I create a dedicated "CC" folder in my inbox with a link that directs all emails on which I am only CC'd directly into the trash folder. I've done this successfully for years (which gave me the nickname of the "guy who never reads his CC emails". I can easily live with that reputation).

The remaining two boxes contain those tasks that are more difficult to resolve.

Box 3 (the *'to delegate'* box) are daily tasks that are not important but urgent. These consist of the multiple daily interruptions, ad-hoc requests, and other distractions that exhaust us after a busy day. A classic example in my own world consists of recurring peer-review requests for biomedical journals. I have multiple simultaneous requests on my desk at any given time. These are 'box 3 issues' with a typical deadline of about 2 weeks for completion. However, if unresolved, these assignments will become urgent and important (box 1) once the assignment has extended beyond its deadline. This should be avoided by all means.

The large bulk of box 3 tasks are possibly best delegated to others (unfortunately, as surgeons we are generally not very good at delegating tasks).

Finally, we reach the most neglected box, number 2 (the *'to plan'* box). This box represents all our projects that are not urgent but are important. You need to think of this as your 'legacy box'. For example, I spent 2 years of my life with intentionally protected time dedicated to box 2 by writing this book. This entails all the things we want to do in our lifetime, but the tasks in the other three boxes won't allow us to address on a given day. The truth is, we tend to push these important (but not urgent) tasks onto the 'tomorrow' back burner, as if tomorrow would be any different than today. And we will keep pushing these important tasks to the next day, into perpetuity.

Remember that 'someday' is not a weekday on your calendar!

There is one simple solution to address this situation: plan every day to dedicate some protected time to the box 2 items. This is where the briefing/debriefing ritual is crucial: to first plan and then review how much time we spent in each of the four boxes at the end of the day, without neglecting box 2.

I realize that trying to get to the important but not urgent plans sounds like *Mission Impossible* considering our busy daily calendars. But it's not. I found an easy and pragmatic solution that has worked for me.

I block out time on my calendar every day — exclusively dedicated to box 2 tasks.

I label the box "THINK" followed by three exclamation marks (see the figure overleaf) to underline the imperative of dedicating time to important but not urgent projects every day. Of note, the only interruptions I tolerate during my protected "THINK" blocks are urgent and important box 1 ad-hoc issues. Needless to say these issues keep interrupting us surgeons every day without advance notice.

November 04, 2014

	4
7 am	**Daily fracture conference** OR conference room
8 00	**3B inpatient ward rounds**
9 00	**Joint Strategy Team: Long Range Strategic Planning** MTG 660 Bannock, 5th Flr, Rm 535, Board Room, FOR EXECUTIVE STAFF ONLY
10 00	**Teleconference Patient Safety in Surgery ed. board;** Call in 1-800-866-5310
	Morgan/Stahel - weekly standing meeting; Dr. Stahel's office; Stahel, Philip F MD
11 00	**THINK!!!**
12 pm	
1 00	
2 00	**Perioperative steering committee meeting** MTG 660 Bannock, 4th floor, Ballroom
3 00	**Patient Safety and Quality Executive Committee meeting** MTG 660 Bannock, 5th Flr, Rm 535, Board Room, FOR EXECUTIVE STAFF ONLY
4 00	
	Microvascular team discussion MTG Pav A, 3rd Flr, Rm A370, Admin. Conf. Rm
5 00	
	City Council Proclamation - S. Thomas 5:30 p.m. City Council Denver City and County Building - City Council Chambers - 1437 Bannock Street - 4th Floor
6 00	
	Humanities Interest Group fundraiser UPI Conference Room, Pavillion for Ethics and Humanities. University of Colorado Medical School
7 00	
8 00	
9 00	

7. Fun

> "Do not get too deeply absorbed in your work to the exclusion of all outside interests. Begin at once some interest other than purely professional."
>
> **Sir William Osler (1849-1919)**

During one of our frequent philosophical discussions, my friend and esteemed colleague Wade Smith once told me: "We should have fun 80% of the time otherwise we must change what we do immediately."

There is wisdom in this statement. Fun seems to go hand-in-hand with optimism and joy; the necessary parts for being a better surgeon.

If we're not enjoying what we do every day, we probably missed our true calling. Fun is important. Businesses know this. They use it to their advantage all the time. Southwest Airlines, for example, is frequently listed as the airline with the lowest staff turnover and highest customer satisfaction rates. Their guiding principle is to exclusively hire qualified people with a good sense of humor. If you've ever traveled on Southwest (personal disclaimer: I don't own any stocks or bonds) you'll understand what I'm talking about. Invariably, the flight attendants are funnier than most stand-up comedians and yet they are excellent at their job. Surgeons should consider taking over the airline's main credo: "Take your job seriously, but not yourself!"

I learned the "work hard, play hard" philosophy from my dear friend, role model and respected surgeon idol Ernest E. ("Gene") Moore. Undoubtedly, Gene is the most accomplished and yet the most modest surgeon I have ever met; clinically, academically, and spiritually. Gene would rather give the rest of the world tribute for his distinguished achievements than to claim any personal credit for his own success.

Needless to say, Gene's also figured out how to have serious fun!

Many years ago, we started a proactive work/life balance venture called "Project Wiesn". The underlying intent was to provide a mental time-out for our surgeons' core group at Denver Health by undertaking a brief 3-day trip from Denver to the Oktoberfest in Munich once a year. Turns out, Gene Moore doesn't just beat me at surgical and academic skills, but also at the number of 'Maß' beers consumed on the Wiesn. And while I've seen many people hung over at Oktoberfest, I've never seen anyone at risk of burnout!

Try to have *fun* every once in a while.

You deserve it.

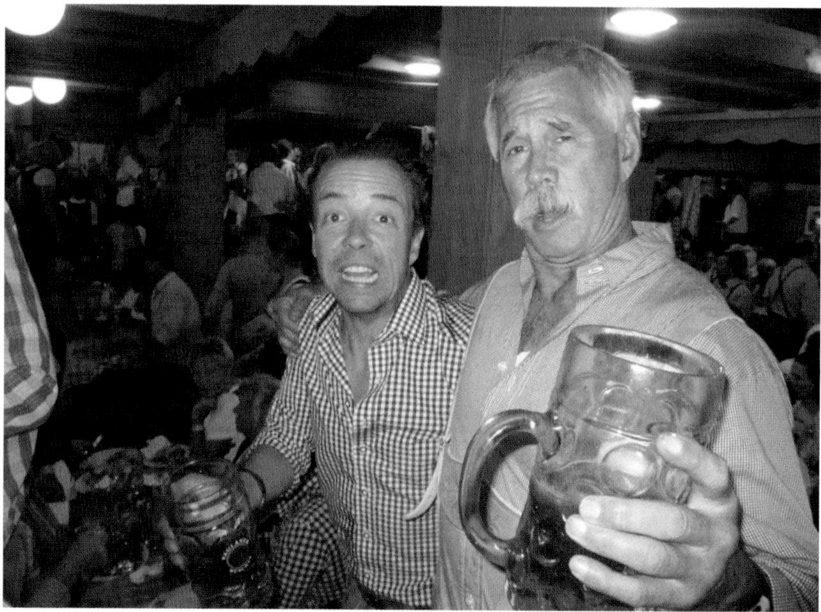

Annually recurring work/life balance restoration project "Wiesn", with my friend Gene Moore (Munich, September 2014).

Chapter 20 What we permit, we promote

"A man does what he must — in spite of personal consequences, in spite of obstacles and dangers and pressures; that is the basis of all human morality."

Sir Winston Churchill (1874-1965)

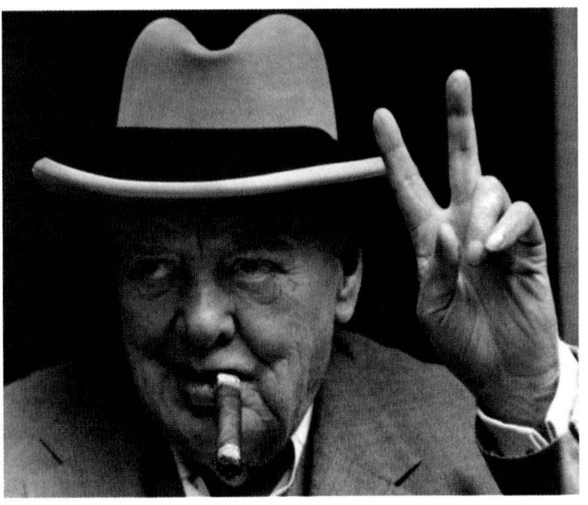

So what have we covered so far?

Complex analytics?

Check.

Statistical calculations?

Check.

Provocative allegations and erratic thoughts based on my own anecdotal experience?

Double check.

So now that you've endured my diatribes for an entire book, I'll address the question you've asked about:

What does it take to become a better surgeon?

The truth is, you're already a good surgeon.

You've trained, worked hard, and dedicated yourself. You've got the technical skills. Just think of the complicated procedures that you perform every day, the elegant and safe art of your work. You've learned how to cut past critical structures, vessels, nerves, and bowels; how to control intra-operative blood loss with the blink of an eye; how to manage your intra-operative complications under any conceivable scenario.

Over the course of your career, you've read hundreds of textbooks and peer-reviewed articles in your field of interest. You continuously improve your knowledge base and technical skillset by attending regular CME courses and hands-on workshops. You know all the surgical indications and contraindications. You've done your work long enough to understand the limits of knowing *when not* to operate. You run a busy surgical practice and you're tremendously respected by your patients, their families, and by your peers.

The truth is, you've finally achieved the ultimate goal: you're known as a 'good and fast' surgeon (I'll admit that's all that I was reaching for as a young resident in training).

You've achieved all it takes.

You've made it.

You're a good surgeon.

But you want to be better...

I recently attended a large workshop on how to improve customer satisfaction in the health care business (isn't it nuts that we call health care a "business" and degrade our patients to "customers"?). The moderator was impressive; he was eloquent and controlled the audience with his dynamic and interactive style. At one point, he asked a straight-up personal question: "When you guys were kids, what did you see yourselves becoming as adults?"

A shouting contest erupted as the audience yelled out a wide range of professional aspirations: "A physician!" — "A surgeon!" — "A paramedic!" — "A fire fighter!" — "A nurse!"

I didn't say anything, though I was impressed with the audience's assertive answers. And, to be honest, I felt a bit embarrassed thinking back on my own limited ambitions when I was a kid. Growing up, I had no idea what I wanted to be as an adult. I certainly never guessed that I'd end up working in a hospital. I never once thought I'd be smart enough go to med school or ambitious and competitive enough to become a surgeon. My childhood dreams were very simple and modest; all my life, I only ever knew that I wanted to be a *servant*.

That sounds silly but it's true.

That's all I still want to be.

I want to serve my community, heal my patients, and mentor my trainees. I want to serve my family and my children by providing them with the love and self-confidence they'll need to master any challenge on this planet. That's it. And that's why I didn't speak up in response to the moderator's question; my childhood ambitions were not nearly as sophisticated and heroic as anyone else's in the audience.

Yet, the 'saints of humanity' have historically embraced my endeavor. Russian novelist Leo Tolstoy (1828-1910) stated unequivocally that: "the sole meaning of life is to serve humanity."

Transposed to our profession, you could summarize this notion more pragmatically by saying that: "the purpose of a surgeon's life is a life of purpose."

Looking for a preventive strategy against burnout? There you go – short and concise. The humanitarian philosopher-scientist Albert Schweitzer (1875-1965) wrote: "I don't know what your destiny will be, but one thing I know: the only ones among you who will be really happy are those who will have sought and found how to serve."

Clearly, being dedicated to a career helping others guided my quest towards becoming a better surgeon. It took me 20 years of *blood, sweat and tears* to get there. Do you want a practical example that relates to my surgical practice?

Fair enough.

I burn through about 100 business cards each week. I hand them out to all my patients and their families, after each encounter. No exception. But contrary to most generic business cards, mine lists my email address and personal cell phone number.

Why?

Because I feel that serving our patient means to be accessible to their needs at any time. I am strongly convinced that this is the only way for patients and families to have 24/7 access to a 'personal friend' inside the hospital. Prior to this insight I used to write my cell phone number on the business card whenever I felt a patient was 'worthy' to give me a call if needed. The Mayor of Denver, the Governor of Colorado, and other selected VIP patients had this distinct honor. Until that insightful moment of truth when I asked myself if I wanted to live the rest of my life as a hypocrite or as a servant?

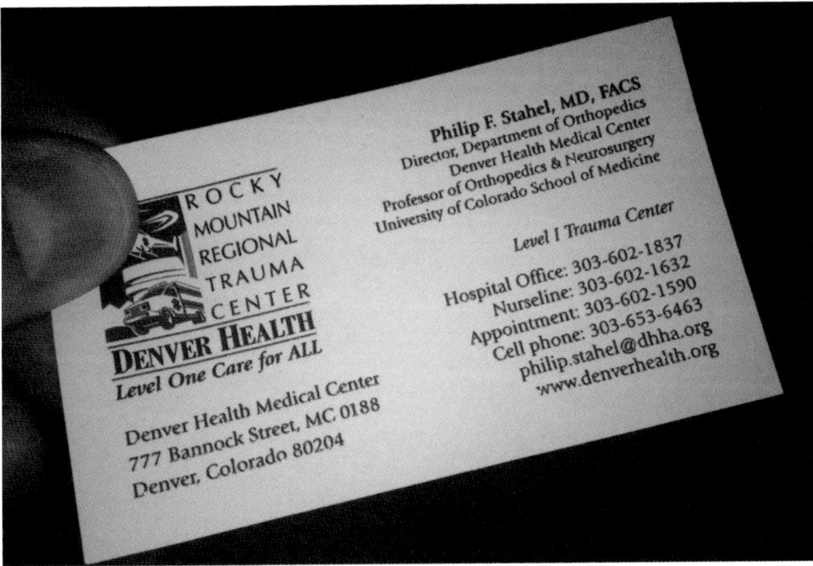

I have certainly been labeled as "crazy" by many of my peers, partners and colleagues. Yet, I actually believe that the decision to be accessible to my patients and their families without restriction, at all times, was the singular tipping point in my attempt to become a better surgeon.

I took a calculated risk (using the formula described in Chapter 7), and I've not regretted it once.

And this, my friends, is the core message I want to send you.

If you live to serve, you will eventually become a leader. You can only be a leader if you're a credible role model 'in the trenches'. And that, very simply, is what I consider to be the singular distinction between a *good* surgeon and a *better* surgeon: better surgeons are *leaders!*

Nothing more, nothing less.

So, how do you recognize a true leader?

Well, have you ever spontaneously picked up litter?

I'm talking about pieces of paper, plastic cups, and candy bar wrappers; the kinds of things we see in the hallways of an office building or a clinic office on a daily basis. The little bits of trash that most people tend to avoid. They'll walk right past, mumbling that someone should be doing a better job cleaning the building. Or they may not even take notice in the first place.

What about you? Do you notice trash? Do you pick it up?

That's the simple unifying characteristic of servants and leaders; we pick up litter because it's the right thing to do (as servants) and to instill this behavior into those who look up to us (as role models and leaders).

Frankly, I'd classify people by three distinct categories based on their habit of picking up litter:

- *Natural born leaders* – people who pick up trash as an instinctual act of kindness and empathy (even when unwitnessed). This rare breed of leaders are driven by 'doing what's right' at all times, and they don't have to be incentivized. These are the 'better surgeons'.
- *Conditional leaders* – people who pick up trash only when there is someone else around to see them do it. These are people who can grow to become leaders by trading the self-serving aspect of their actions towards becoming true servants. These are 'good surgeons' on the path to becoming better.
- *'The rest'* are the large bulk of people who never pick up litter, regardless of whether someone is watching. It's hard to imagine that surgeons in this category would ever grow beyond the walls of their own ego.

By the way, there is, of course, a fourth category — our janitors. People who pick up other people's trash for a living; they are truly the *world's eternal servants*.

You're not going to believe this but here's one of my habits. I love making a game of picking up litter. The rules are simple; find a plastic bag on the street as your first 'trash trophy', then fill it up with random litter. You can rest assured that by the time the bag is full I'll walk into the next plastic bag to be filled up, too. This can easily become an endless game. For me, I stop when: a) I can't carry any more bags; or b) I make it to a trash can, whichever comes first. I'm a champion at the sport.

All kidding aside, the concept of personal accountability for hand hygiene is essentially the same as that of picking up litter.

Just remember the classic quote from the leadership world: "What we permit, we promote."

ROAD TRASH WARRIORS
Picking up the Planet's
Road Trash
One Mile at a Time

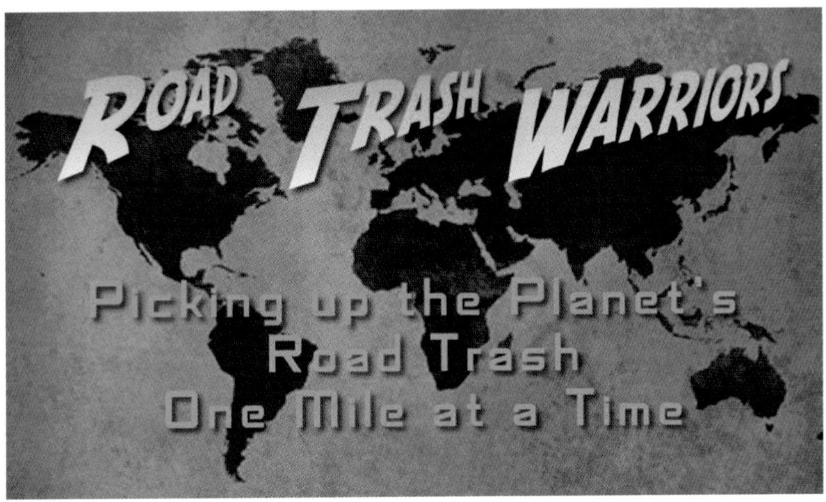

If you walk past litter on the street, your action implies that it's OK to pollute. If you don't stop and reprimand staff for walking into a patient's room without washing their hands, you send a clear message to those who look up to you that: "It's OK not to wash your hands occasionally, because our leader obviously tolerates it."

This is why leaders have to be tough, not just popular.

When it comes to keeping our patients safe, we must be tough, decisive, and uncompromising. Here's another quote for unwavering leadership: "Never apologize for setting high expectations!"

For me, the best textbook definition of a 'better surgeon' is derived from the legendary NASA Flight Director, Gene Kranz (who many readers may remember from the brilliant portrayal by Ed Harris in the blockbuster *Apollo 13*).

On January 27, 1967, a flash fire swept through the Apollo 1 command module during a launch rehearsal and killed all three astronauts. In the wake of this catastrophe that would subsequently change NASA safety protocols and ensure Apollo 11's successful lunar mission, Gene Kranz said:

> "From this day forward, Flight Control will be known by two words: tough & competent. Tough means that we are forever accountable for what we do or what we fail to do. We will never again compromise our responsibilities. Competent means we will never take anything for granted. We will never be found short in our knowledge and in our skills."

There you go: "tough & competent" are the mandatory ingredients for achieving the goal postulated in the title of this book.

If you're *competent*, you're good.

It takes the *tough leadership* aspect to allow you to become a better surgeon.

And let me be clear: you don't have to hold a professor title to be a leader. A junior resident can easily assume a leadership role by holding interns and medical students accountable for core measures, such as perfect handovers and uncompromising hand hygiene. A private practice surgeon can be a leader to his partners and his team by living up to the highest ethical standards of our profession.

It's all in your credibility as a role model.

To me, "tough & competent" implies to never ask for permission for doing the right thing and to hold our teams accountable for their actions, whether our decisions are popular or not. Remember that not every popular decision is right, and not every right decision is popular.

That's credible leadership; "to walk the walk" and not just "talk the talk":

- To wash our hands before and after entering a patient's room.
- To pick up litter when we see it.
- To know each team member's name throughout the organization, including the janitors' names.
- To go by first name with everyone in the hospital.
- To lead by example, and not by intimidation.

As Albert Camus (1913-1960), the French Nobel Prize winning philosopher, correctly stated: "Nothing is more despicable than respect based on fear."

In my own practice, I have applied an unconventional approach towards eradicating the risk of intimidation associated with the use of academic titles. I simply go by my first name with every member of the team. It took months and years of convincing our nurses and house staff that I am to be addressed as "Phil", not "Doctor", "Sir", or "Professor".

This ordinary approach works.

Seriously. Try it out.

Not only does using first names drop hierarchy but it also allows for team building driven by mutual trust and respect. Most importantly, this aborts the 'phantom menace' of a surgeon's sense of entitlement and the associated dangers previously discussed in the book.

Let's be honest, I didn't invent this concept. This is actually standard in many other high-risk industries, including professional aviation. Going by first names in the cockpit keeps planes safe. Similarly, allowing a nurse to speak up in the OR has certainly kept my patients safe on multiple, uncounted occasions. For the simple reason that it's much easier for a scrub tech to stop me from causing harm to a patient by saying: "Hey Phil, what the (expletive) are you doing?!"

In his bestselling book *Outliers*,[69] Malcolm Gladwell described a senior captain's approach to attenuating his co-pilot's fear of speaking up like this:

> "On a very simple level, one of the things we insist upon at my airline is that the first officer and the captain call each other by their first names. We think that helps. It's just harder to say 'Captain, you're doing something wrong' than to use a name. One thing I personally try to do, is to put myself a little down. I say to my co-pilots: 'I don't fly very often. Three or four times a month. You fly a lot more. If you see me doing something stupid, it's because I don't fly very often. So tell me. Help me out.' Hopefully, that helps them to speak up."

Could you imagine extrapolating this to the OR?

Well, guess what? It works for me.

The truth can be boiled down to a simple fact: if we're wholeheartedly determined to become *better surgeons*, we have to be able to lock up our egos.

---

[69] Gladwell M. *Outliers - The Story of Success.* New York, USA: Back Bay Books, 2008.

Be modest. Be empathetic.

Under-promise and over-deliver!

So you say you want to be a better surgeon?

Pick up the next piece of litter you come across.

The world will thank you.

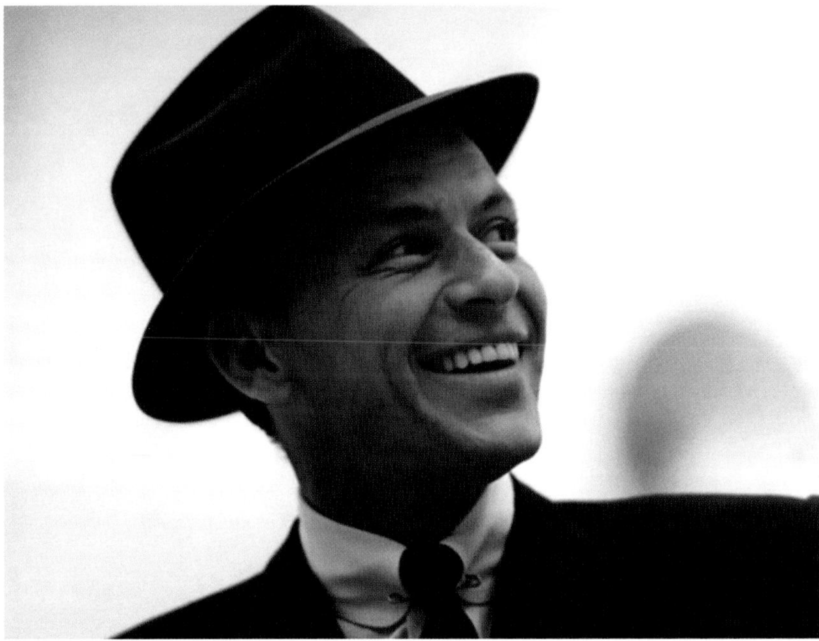

"Regrets, I've had a few, but then again, too few to mention..." Frank Sinatra (1915-1998).

Epilogue

By Wade Smith, MD [70]

Blood, Sweat & Tears masquerades as a book about becoming a better surgeon. In truth, this is the story of becoming a better human. Contrary to the plethora of 'tell all' books exposing the seamy underbelly of medicine or any other entity that is supposed to do good but sometimes does not, this is *a tale of truth and hope*.

Phil Stahel describes with great personal detail what happens when men and women strive to do their best and yet discover that this is not always good enough. From personal failure to patient tragedies to epiphany, this book reads like a classic redemption novel, except that every bit of it is true.

Surgery is a tricky business requiring long training, dedication, a bit of megalomania and a focus on technical details in order to be competent. As Phil Stahel discovers in the course of his work, and describes to us, going beyond competence takes insight and personal qualities that do not naturally occur in surgical training. Empathy, humility and caring for others does not come automatically. The author admits that these qualities increasingly became important to him through participating and witnessing the devastating effects of surgical complications on patients' lives.

We have all been there.

Every one of us who has practiced surgery knows the feeling of talking to a patient's family after things did not go well, driving home alone from

---

[70] Wade Smith is a senior orthopaedic surgeon practicing in Denver, Colorado, and co-founding editor of the open-access, peer-reviewed journal *Patient Safety in Surgery*.

the hospital in guilt, knowing that we could have done better. We all have *blood, sweat and tears* on our hands and yet, for many of us, these terrible experiences do not lead to growth and insight.

And that is why this book is so important.

Phil Stahel saw what many of us have not. He saw the tragedy of medical care when it is not focused on the patient and rather on other aspects including finances, market competition, or 'doctor ego'. He saw this and presents the pathway he walked, which we can learn from. More importantly, he provides insights on how to shorten the learning curve to get to that point of caring and to improved patient outcomes without leaving a 'trail of the wounded'. This task requires significant effort, including keeping track of complications, scheduling adequate time to talk to patients about their surgery, and being willing to admit mistakes.

How many of us are truly committed to change for the sake of our patients' wellbeing?

Blood, Sweat & Tears is a great book, one of a kind, and destined to be a medical classic. What makes the book exceptional is the narrative about a difficult human endeavor, often done imperfectly, by humans who have been told they should be 'perfect'. This quintessential paradox is why this book is a practical story about life and will likely be of interest and enjoyment to many outside the realm of medicine.

I have had the privilege of knowing and working with the author for many years and I can vouch for the reality of his experiences and the truth of his conclusions.

Phil really does pick up trash when he goes for a run; and so should we all.

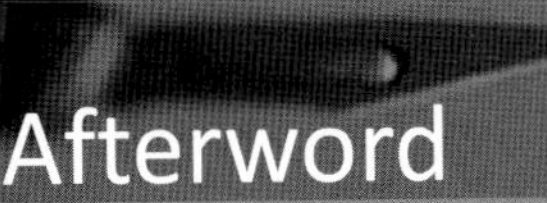

Afterword

By Ted J. Clarke, MD [71]

The life of a surgeon is difficult. Life- and limb-threatening problems do not necessarily occur at convenient times. Surgery is not for the weak as it requires physical strength, emotional stamina, and unquenchable intellectual curiosity. Underneath these prerequisites lies the most important of all surgical requirements: the patient. With his emphasis on patient care found through empathy, shared decision-making, and attention to detail, Phil Stahel is telling the surgeon of today and tomorrow about the way to quality improvement and self-fulfillment.

Blood, Sweat & Tears charts the path for the surgeon's journey to excellence. In part, Phil sets this journey by using a seemingly endless list of quotes that draw from the wisdom and experiences of leaders from multiple fields. The thoughts of William Osler, "Listen to the patient – he is telling you the diagnosis", come through loud and clear when Sir William is seemingly staring at the reader. Intermixed with the wisdom of yesteryear are notions that clearly play out today. As his colleague Wade Smith observed: "If we are not having fun 80% of the time, we need to look for a new profession." By drawing on the wit and wisdom of Sesame Street characters, Sherlock Holmes, Alfred Hitchcock and more, Phil Stahel is clearly having fun with his book. The reader should enjoy such insights.

The need for ongoing surgical quality improvement resonates throughout the book. Whether it is simple hand washing before and after patient encounters or personal data collection of surgeries performed, the

[71] Ted Clarke is a retired orthopaedic surgeon, renowned patient safety advocate, and CEO and Chairman of COPIC, the largest physician insurance company in Colorado.

reader continually learns that there is no substitute for ongoing adherence to improvement in patient care. The "$20 challenge" that is issued to medical students for observing non-compliance in hand washing exemplifies the importance of adhering to known protocols that work. How can the meat industry do a better job at policing its workers than our surgical colleagues do? This conundrum ranks as a mystery that Phil Stahel clearly will not tolerate. The reader senses that like the comic character Pogo, he is telling us, "We have met the enemy, and he is us."

AH, POGO, THE BEAUTY OF THE FOREST PRIMEVAL GETS ME IN THE HEART.
IT GETS ME IN THE FEET, PORKYPINE.
2TH DAY 1971
PUBLISHERS-HALL SYNDICATE, INC.
IT IS HARD WALKIN' ON THIS STUFF.
YEP, SON, WE HAVE MET THE ENEMY AND HE IS US.

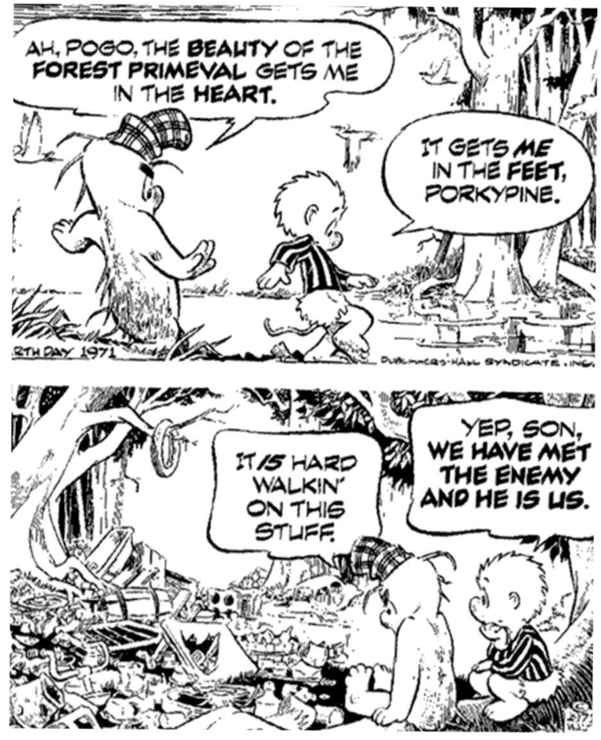

Data collection clearly underlies surgical quality improvement, and represents a missing part in the ongoing development of many practicing surgeons. How many surgeons know their own results when talking about the odds, probability, and risk of a particular procedure that is being suggested to the patient? We all too often fall back upon a recent article or a multi-center study that showed an infection rate of X or a bleeding rate of Y. Although the literature provides important benchmarks for surgery, unless we were participants in the study, such 'facts' do not reflect our own experiences. Certainly, our patients want to know the experience of the surgeon who is about to do their case. The personal stories of Michael Skolnik, Suzie Davis Ingraham, and others emphasize the importance of sharing honest information with the patient — an essential partner in the surgical experience.

Phil Stahel recognizes that surgery is a most challenging way of life, but he compares our rewards and compensations with other challenging jobs. The detailed wages of meat packers and coal miners emphasize society's remunerations for our work. With such rewards comes responsibility, and it is clear that the expectations for surgeons are and should be at the highest level. That is why honest reflections and reviews of our work are so important and why surgeons must be intimately involved in this process. Yes, various systems can create barriers for patient care, but the surgeon must find ways to overcome such impediments. Ownership of our patients' outcomes is essential to success, and it is clear that various regulations and restrictions imposed by hospitals, health plans, legislatures, and others can work against the patient's best interest. "Always, always put the patient first" is a mantra that is chanted throughout the book.

The challenges of a surgeon's life can lead to a variety of personal failures.

An awareness of burnout with its many symptoms may help create a path for salvation for the surgeon and/or his colleague. Encouraging other interests and allowing for important relationships with family and friends offers some mitigation for this problem. Finding joy in your work and your patients offers another means of avoiding career dissatisfaction.

The training of a surgeon involves observation, oversight, practice, repetition, and eventually proficiency. The great majority of surgical training revolves around the development of technical skills and procedural judgment. Hopefully, judgment is part of training as we learn the what, when, where, and why to do a particular procedure. Equally important in this training mix of surgery is a variety of 'nots': why not, where not, when not, and how not.

The emphasis on *empathy* is a crucial but neglected part of quality improvement. Why do our patients so frequently not adhere to our instructions? Putting yourself in the patient's position creates an essential surgeon-patient bond that underlies an optimal outcome. Phil did not write the golden rule of "love thy neighbor as thyself", but it is clear that he sees this as an essential part of the surgeon-patient partnership. Both surgeon and patient will feel this effect, and it will pay dividends for both parties in the near and distant future.

It is an important but disturbing reflection that many medical students lose their empathetic qualities during their clerkship years. There are many reasons that underlie this loss including our role models, the frantic pace of clinical activities, and the lack of clear direction as to the medical student role. Importantly, Phil gives us a path to finding our empathy by rediscovering our humanism. Relating to the janitor, the nurse, and other members of the care team as people is an important first step in understanding the common ground that we share with our patients. Letting each member of the surgical team call the professor by his first name clearly tells the staff that all are important and essential. Giving his phone number to his patients shows the trust that Phil shares with those who trust him.

The final section on the spiritual surgeon brings new thoughts to our profession. The servant surgeon knows his role is to serve his patient, his friend. He understands that he has been entrusted with a special role for our community, and it is his duty to assure the best outcome for each and every patient. Such an obligation is an ongoing commitment to surgical education, data collection and analysis, and quality improvement. The story of the surgeon's journey goes beyond the operating room. It is a story where the clinic, the emergency room, and the hospital ward are given equal prominence in the development of a successful surgeon.

As I reflect upon my own 35-year career in surgery, I remember the eagerness with which I first approached operating room days. "A chance to cut is a chance to cure" and "the only way to heal is with cold steel" were chants that my fellow residents and I would often repeat. The operating room was its own sanctuary away from many realities of patient care. With time, I have learned to appreciate other parts of patient care. In the clinic, I have a chance to know the patient as a person, and I have an opportunity to educate the patient as I would want to be educated.

My path to becoming a better surgeon is far from over but my time to accomplish this is short. I truly wish that I had read such a book many decades ago as I began my life in surgery, but back then no such work was available. With *Blood, Sweat & Tears*, Phil Stahel has directed me to some needed tools that might help me reach this laudatory goal of ongoing quality improvement. I am most appreciative for his reflections and observations, and I remain hopeful that perhaps someday I might become a better surgeon.

Acknowledgments

First and foremost, I am indebted to my publisher Nikki Bramhill for her trust and support of a project by a guy who doesn't answer his emails.

I would also like to thank all my friends and colleagues who took the time to read and correct the multiple drafts of the book.

I must acknowledge my friends Keith Breese, Marc Pinto and Kim Spahn for their endless efforts engaged in a Don Quixotesque task of helping me turn my incomprehensible initial drafts ("What did you mean when you wrote that?") into artistic narrative content. Keith, Marc and Kim are the 'secret editors' behind this book.

My sincere gratitude goes to Marty Makary, Wade Smith, and Ted Clarke for dedicating their time and expertise to contributing the foreword, epilogue and afterword.

I am furthermore indebted to my friends and esteemed colleagues Jeff Johnson and Jerry Buckley for reviewing the book from the surgeon's perspective.

Special thanks to my dear friend and spiritual mentor Elizabeth Tadikonda for providing critical feedback on the spiritual surgeon section, and to Nicole Morgan and Barbara Butler for volunteering as 'guinea pig' test readers of the book.

My gratitude also goes to Julie Lonborg and Scott Dressel-Martin for providing the book cover image and stock photos from the Denver Health picture archive, and to 'BigZ' Felix Zindel and Yohan Robinson for contributing images to the chapter on resident training.

I also want to acknowledge my respected friend José Santiago for critical review of the manuscript and for contributing the 'coffee cup story' to the burnout chapter.

My sincere gratitude goes to my friend and patient advocate Patty Skolnik for sharing the horrific story of her only son Michael's preventable death secondary to unnecessary surgery. I have yet to meet a single reader who was not moved by Michael's heartbreaking story described in the chapter "Nothing about me, without me!"

I am also indebted to my dear friends and respected physician role models of equanimity and compassionate patient-centered care, Phil Mehler and Patty Gabow, and to my surgeon idols and world-renowned masters of trauma surgery, Ernest E. ('Gene') Moore and Otmar Trentz.

This book is furthermore dedicated to my 'brothers in arms' who sacrifice their lives and careers to doing the right thing for their patients at all times:

Todd VanderHeiden, Christoph Heyde, Thilo John, Hannes Fakler, Rich Schulick, Andy Meacham, Abraham Nussbaum, and all my surgeon friends and partners at the Gun & Knife Club at Denver Health.

I am furthermore indebted to my dear friends, research mentors, and Jedi Masters of neurocomplementology, Scott Barnum and Mike Holers.

Sebastian Weckbach deserves credit as the fearless organizer of the annually recurring Wiesn trip to Munich for 'Team USA' — arguably the most effective remedy against surgeon burnout.

I also want to thank my life-long friend of 35 years (and counting), Edgar 'Ede' Landgraf, for always busting my balls — you made me a better person, brother!

My unspoken respect goes to my janitor friends at Denver Health, David Frein and Mike McClain, the true heroes of our society. Thanks for all your hard work in keeping our planet clean!

Thanks to Elvis Presley and Frank Sinatra for providing the soundtrack of my life.

Finally, my deepest gratitude goes to my family:

To Vanessa, Vincent and Cedric, the most 'peculiar' children on this planet (thanks for amazing me every single day!), and to my beautiful wife Aimée. Last but not least, I feel obliged to recognize the epic Mr. Hector for being the most spiritual creature on four legs.

You guys are the core and heart of everything.

Thanks for your unconditional love.

Abbreviations

ACGME	Accreditation Council for Graduate Medical Education
APPAC	Appendicitis Acuta (multicenter, open-label, noninferiority randomized clinical trial)
AWMF	Arbeitsgemeinschaft der Wissenschaftlichen Medizinischen Fachgesellschaften
CAPCOM	Capsule Communicator (NASA)
CBC	Complete blood count
CDC	Centers for Disease Control and Prevention
CEO	Chief Executive Officer
CFO	Chief Financial Officer
CME	Continuing medical education
COPIC	Colorado Physician Insurance Company
CRASH	Corticosteroid Randomization after Significant Head Injury
CT	Computed tomography
DVT	Deep venous thrombosis
EBM	Evidence-based medicine
ECG	Electrocardiogram
ED	Emergency department
EEG	Electroencephalogram
EHR	Electronic health record
EMT	Emergency medicine technician
ER	Emergency room
FAA	Federal Aviation Administration

FARC	Fuerzas Armadas Revolucionarias de Colombia
FIDELITY	Finnish Degenerative Meniscal Lesion Study
HCAHPS	Hospital Consumer Assessment of Healthcare Providers and Systems
H&P	History and physical examination
ICU	Intensive care unit
IOM	Institute of Medicine
ISI	Institute for Scientific Information
MIA	Missing in action
M&M	Morbidity and mortality
MRI	Magnetic resonance imaging
MRSA	Methicillin-resistant *Staphylococcus aureus*
NASA	National Aeronautics and Space Administration
NASCIS	National Acute Spinal Cord Injury Study
NIH	National Institutes of Health
NP	Nurse practitioner
OR	Operating room
PA	Physician assistant
PACS	Picture archiving and communication system
PE	Pulmonary embolism
PGY	Postgraduate year
POD	Postoperative day
Q&A	Questions and Answers
QA	Quality assurance
QI	Quality improvement
RTL	Radio Television Luxembourg
RVU	Relative Value Unit
SUV	Sport utility vehicle
WHO	World Health Organization

Glossary

Abscess

An abscess is an enclosed collection of liquefied tissue as a host-derived white blood cell reaction against invading pathogens (also known as "pus" in lay terminology).

Anastomosis

Surgical restoration of the lumen between two tubular structures (e.g. vessels, bowels, etc.)

Aphasia

The loss of a previously held ability to speak or understand spoken or written language, due to disease or injury of the brain.

Arthrotomy

Incision into a joint.

Cholecystectomy

Surgical removal of the gallbladder.

Deep venous thrombosis

A condition in which a blood clot forms in a vein deep beneath the skin, typically in the leg or pelvic area.

Disseminated intravascular coagulation

A hemorrhagic disorder that occurs following the uncontrolled activation of clotting factors and fibrinolytic enzymes throughout small blood vessels, resulting in tissue necrosis and bleeding.

Electrocardiogram (EKG, ECG)

The graphic record produced by an electrocardiograph.

Electroencephalogram (EEG)

A graphic record produced by an electroencephalograph.

Hemiparalysis

Paralysis of one side of the body.

Hydrocephalus

Hydrocephalus is an abnormal expansion of cavities (ventricles) within the brain that is caused by the accumulation of cerebrospinal fluid. Hydrocephalus comes from two Greek words: *hydros* means water and *cephalus* means head.

Knee scope

Surgical slang for knee arthroscopy.

Laparoscopic cholecystectomy

Minimally-invasive surgical removal of the gallbladder through small buttonhole incisions in the abdominal cavity (also known as "lap chole" in surgical slang).

Laparotomy

Incision through the abdominal wall.

Laps

A compress consisting of several layers of gauze used for packing and protection of visceral organs during a laparotomy (surgical slang term for "laparotomy sponges").

Meniscectomy

Partial or complete surgical excision of one of the two crescent-shaped cartilage buffers of the knee joint (meniscus).

Meniscus

A crescent-shaped fibrocartilaginous structure of the knee and the acromioclavicular, sternoclavicular, and temporomandibular joints.

Metastasis

A malignant tumor growth or deposit that has spread via lymph or blood to an area of the body remote from the primary tumor.

Multiple organ failure

A progressive condition usually characterized by the combined failure of several organs such as the lungs, liver, kidney, along with some clotting mechanisms.

OR bridge

The generic designation for the 'command center' of the operating rooms.

Psychosis

A mental disorder characterized by symptoms, such as delusions or hallucinations, that indicate impaired contact with reality.

Pulmonary embolism

Embolism of pulmonary arteries, most frequently by detached fragments of thrombus from a leg or pelvic vein.

Respiratory arrest

The cessation of breathing.

Sepsis

Sepsis is a potentially life-threatening complication of an infection that occurs when bacteria and chemicals released into the bloodstream to fight the infection trigger a systemic inflammatory response throughout the body. This inflammation can trigger a cascade of changes that may lead to multiple organ failure. If sepsis progresses to septic shock, blood pressure drops dramatically, which may lead to death.

Septic arthritis

An acute form of arthritis characterized by bacterial inflammation of a joint caused by the spread of bacteria through the bloodstream from an infection elsewhere in the body or by contamination of a joint during trauma or surgery.

Thalamic chronic pain syndrome

Synonym: "central pain syndrome". This is a chronic neurological disorder caused by damage to the central nervous system after various insults, including stroke, brain tumors, and trauma. Common symptoms include pain in the face, arms and/or legs. Pain is often constant and can be severe in intensity. Affected individuals are hypersensitive to painful stimuli. In severe cases, the pain can be agonizing, unrelenting and dramatically affect a person's quality of life.

Whipple procedure

The removal of part or all of the pancreas, duodenum, proximal jejunum, distal stomach, and common bile duct for the surgical treatment of pancreatic cancer.

Image copyright

Disclosure:

The author (P.F.S.) owns the copyright on all images, tables and graphs used in this book with the exception of the items listed below. Reprint permission for all other sources are outlined below.

Title page & back cover	**Surgeon walking into the OR.** © Scott Dressel-Martin & Julie Lonborg, Denver Health Archive, 2015.
The author, pv	**Philip F. Stahel, MD, FACS.** © Scott Dressel-Martin & Julie Lonborg, Denver Health Archive, 2015.
Chapter 2, p11	**Bedside empathetic physician.** © Scott Dressel-Martin & Julie Lonborg, Denver Health Archive, 2015.
Chapter 3, p21	**The Hulk stamp.** iStock/Getty Images, ID 20708910, © by Ken Brown (July 5, 2012).
Chapter 4, p33	**Sir William Osler (1849-1919), Canadian physician, aged 63.** L0074448, © Wellcome Library, London. Photograph c. 1912. From: PP/WRO, Professor Oliver Wrong. Collection: Archives & Manuscripts. Library reference no.: Archives and Manuscripts PP/WRO.

Chapter 4, p39 **TV cartoon.**
iStock/Getty Images, ID 53372292, © by Frank Ramspott (December 4, 2014).

Chapter 6, p47 **Craps dice.**
iStock/Getty Images, ID 12212561, © by mphillips007 (March 7, 2010).

Chapter 7, p51 **Businesswoman balancing over sharks.**
iStock/Getty Images, ID 50198946, © by CreativaImages (November 2, 2014).

Chapter 7, p53 **Newspaper, terrorism alert.**
iStock/Getty Images, ID 10634215, © by gmutlu (September 28, 2009).

Chapter 7, p54 **African continent graph.**
© tfm publishing Ltd., 2016.

Chapter 8, p61 **Newspaper, Ebola outbreak.**
iStock/Getty Images, ID 49026166, © by Kirby Hamilton (October 8, 2014).

Chapter 8, p66 **ATLS student manual, 9th ed.**
Reprinted with permission, © American College of Surgeons, 2012.

Chapter 8, p68 **Table 1. Overview on the 12 selected peer-reviewed journals analyzed in our study.**
Reprinted with permission from: Hasenboehler E, *et al.* Bias towards publishing positive results in orthopedic and general surgery: a patient safety issue? *Patient Saf Surg* 2007; 1: 4.
Open access, Creative Commons Attribution License.
© by Hasenboehler *et al*, 2007.

Chapter 9, p71 **Doctor head-in-the-sand.**
iStock/Getty Images, ID 24050526, © by marvinh (May 10, 2013).

Chapter 9, p78 **Reported events per attending surgeon, shown as percentages (number of events per 100 surgical procedures), during the pre-implementation and post-implementation phases of the new QA process (A) and grading of occurrences after weekly peer review, shown as occurrences per 100 surgical procedures for the entire department (B).**
Reprinted with permission from: Stahel PF, *et al.* Disclosure and reporting of surgical complications — a double-edged sword? *Am J Med Qual* 2010; 25: 398-402.
© SAGE Publications Inc., 2010.

Chapter 10, p79 **Hand hygiene.**
© Scott Dressel-Martin & Julie Lonborg, Denver Health Archive, 2015.

Chapter 10, p86 **Siberian coal miners.**
© Jacob Ehrbahn/POLFOTO/PA Images.

Chapter 10, p92 **The Hawthorne Works, Cicero, IL (1925).**
This image is in the public domain.
Western Electric Company.

Chapter 10, p93 **Unit floor plan and location of real-time location system components.**
Reprinted with permission from: Srigley JA, *et al.* Quantification of the Hawthorne effect in hand hygiene compliance monitoring using an electronic monitoring system: a retrospective cohort study. *BMJ Quality & Safety* 2014; 23: 974-80.
Open access, Creative Commons Attribution License.
© BMJ Publishing Group Ltd., 2014.

Chapter 10, p94 **Meat packing.**
iStock/Getty Images, ID 57054146, © by Pilin_Petunyia (February 1, 2015).

Chapter 11, p101 **Eat-what-you-kill cartoon.**
iStock/Getty Images, ID 14152146, © by antonbrand (September 7, 2010).

Chapter 12, p117 **Michael Skolnik (March 15, 1979 — June 4, 2004).**
Reprinted with permission, © Patty Skolnik.

Chapter 12, p120 **Michael Skolnik with his mother Patty at the bedside on the first night after his intraventricular drain had been placed.**
Reprinted with permission, © Patty Skolnik.

Chapter 13, p127 **Mountaineer team.**
iStock/Getty Images, ID 50369436, © by vm (October 27, 2014).

Chapter 13, p132 **Suzannah "Suzie" Davis Ingraham (December 10, 1977 — July 3, 2010).**
Reprinted with permission, © Marc Pinto, 2009.

Chapter 13, p138 **Three Musketeers.**
iStock/Getty Images, ID 17485473, © by Verzh (August 24, 2011).

Chapter 13, p140 **Rehab checklist.**
Reprinted with permission, © Marc Pinto, 2015.

Chapter 13, p142 **Marc Pinto on crutches.**
Reprinted with permission, © Marc Pinto, 2015.

Chapter 14, p143 **Clinic patient encounter.**
© Scott Dressel-Martin & Julie Lonborg, Denver Health Archive, 2015.

Chapter 14, p152 **Patient marking wrist.**
Reprinted with permission, © Kyros Ipaktchi, 2015.

Chapter 14, p154 **Arsonist.**
iStock/Getty Images, ID 17181263, © by James Brey (July 21, 2011).

Chapter 16, p163 **RMS Titanic departing Southampton on April 10, 1912.**
F.G.O. Stuart (1843-1923).
This image is in the public domain.

Chapter 16, p165 **Human error contribution in collision and grounding of oil tankers.**
Reprinted with permission from: Martins MR, Maturana MC. Human error contribution in collision and grounding of oil tankers. *Risk Analysis* 2010; 30: 674-98.
© John Wiley and Sons, 2010.

Chapter 16, p170 **Wrong-patient and wrong-site surgery occurrences in Colorado before and after implementation of the "Universal Protocol" on July 1, 2014.**
Reprinted with permission from: Stahel PF, *et al.* Wrong-site and wrong-patient procedures in the Universal Protocol era: analysis of a prospective database of physician self-reported occurrences. *Arch Surg* 2010; 145: 978-84.
© American Medical Association, 2010.

Chapter 16, p171 **Table 7. Results from our study reflecting the extent of patient harm from wrong-patient and wrong-site surgical procedures.**
Reprinted with permission from: Stahel PF, *et al.* Wrong-site and wrong-patient procedures in the Universal Protocol era: analysis of a prospective database of physician self-reported occurrences. *Arch Surg* 2010; 145: 978-84.
© American Medical Association, 2010.

Chapter 16, p175 **Rocket launch.**
iStock/Getty Images, ID 13592459, © by deslover (July 18, 2010).

Chapter 16, p178 **Cockpit.**
iStock/Getty Images, ID 49147760, © by Matus Duda (October 16, 2014).

Chapter 17, p181 **Cartoon.**
Reprinted with permission, © BigZ, Felix Zindel, Switzerland.

Chapter 17, p184 **Fatigue, alcohol and performance impairment.**
Reprinted with permission from: Dawson D, Reid K. Fatigue, alcohol and performance impairment. *Nature* 1997; 388: 235.
© Nature Publishing Group, 1997.

Chapter 17, p188 **Yohan Robinson EEG monitoring.**
Reprinted with permission, © Yohan Robinson.

Chapter 18, p195 **Time running out.**
iStock/Getty Images, ID 56348146, © by sezer66 (January 21, 2015).

Chapter 18, p197 **Doctor running.**
iStock/Getty Images, ID 17519261, © by leaf (August 30, 2011).

Chapter 18, p203 **Janitor Mike McClain.**
© Scott Dressel-Martin & Julie Lonborg, Denver Health Archive, 2015.

Chapter 20, p239 **Road Trash Warriors.**
Reprinted with permission.
© Road Trash Warriors, 2009.
http://roadtrashwarriors.org.

Afterword, p248 **Pogo daily strip from *Earth Day*, 1971.**
A 1971 Earth Day comic strip written and illustrated by Walt Kelly, featuring Pogo and Porkypine. Reprinted with permission.
© OGPI, 1971.

Index

accessibility 236-7
accountability 81-5, 164, 249
  hand hygiene 89-94, 239-40
adverse events 72
  see also complication rates; medical errors
advocacy for the patient 128-37
Africa, a big place 54
allergies to medicines 134, 151
amputation, avoiding 145-6
analgesic overdose 12-14
ankle fractures, unnecessary removal of screws 104-6
aortic anastomosis, leaking 4-10
APPAC trial (appendectomy) 109
appendectomy 108-9
Aristotle 84, 222
aviation industry 160, 161, 177-9, 209, 231, 242
avoidable surgery 101-16, 147-8
  amputation 145-6
  ankle fixation screw removal 104-6
  appendectomy 108-9
  arthroscopic meniscectomy 106-8
  colloid cyst removal 118-21
  for financial motives 110, 114-16
  Funktionslust 111-13
  for reputational motives 113-14

awareness 222-3

Barton, Clara 117
Bayesian theory (conditional probability) 61-4
bias
 observation bias 92-3
 publication bias 67-9
Biedermann und die Brandstifter (Frisch) 153-4
Blair, Tony 55
blame and shame culture 74-5, 84, 108, 158-62
brain surgery 118-21
briefing/debriefing daily 219
burnout 206, 249
 depression 206, 209
 how to avoid 216-32
 overwork 207-8, 209-11
 threat of litigation 212-16
Bush, George H.W. 224
business cards 236-7

Camus, Albert 241
cancer, terminal 133-7
cardiovascular disease 56
Carlyle, Thomas 225
Carson, Benjamin 51, 57-8
Challenger disaster 174-5
checklists 169-79
Churchill, Sir Winston 36, 81, 233
Citizens for Patient Safety 122
Clarke, Ted 168
clinical trial enrolment 134-5
Clostridium difficile 90
coal miners' working conditions 86
Coelho, Pablo 220

colloid cysts 118-21
communication skills
honesty 42-6
improving 36-8
listening to the patient 33-40, 128, 150-1
questioning the surgeon 128, 144-54
shared decision-making 118-25
compassion 26-7
see also empathy
compassion fatigue 204
complication rates
compilation of data 71-8, 248-9
postoperative infections 89-90, 103
telling the patient 42-4, 152-3
Conan Doyle, Arthur 41, 79
conditional probability 61-4
consent 50, 120
continuity of care, lack of xi, 190-1
COPIC Insurance 168-9

daily rituals 218-20
decision fatigue 60
decision-making
decisiveness 225
and risk 52-8
shared 118-25
defensive medicine 160, 212-13
deference towards surgeons 128-9, 241-2
asking questions 144-54
delegation 228-9
depression 206, 209
detached empathy 18-19
diagnosis 153
discipline 218-20

diuretics, inappropriate use 159
documentation 36, 214, 215

"eat-what-you-kill" phenomenon 115
Ebola, risk of catching 61-4
Edge (The Third Culture) 69
education, medical 249-50
    empathy 25, 28, 250
    work-hour restrictions 182-90
Einstein, Albert 47
Eisenhower, Dwight D. 226, 227
Electronic Health Records (EHRs) 36
email management viii, 228
empathy (or its absence) 17-29
    avoiding burnout 224
    in children 20-2
    definition 17-19
    marker of 201-2
    in the medical profession 15, 18-19, 22-9, 137, 203-4, 250
entitlement in surgeons 196-200, 242
evidence-based medicine (EBM) 65-70
expected utility theory 60
experts 64, 135

fail-safes 161
family members as advocates 130
FIDELITY trial (partial meniscectomy) 107-8
financial incentives for unnecessary surgery 110, 114-16
Franklin, Benjamin 55
fraudulent surgery 110
Frein, David 87, 88, 202
Fukushima Daiichi accident 56
fun 231-2
Funktionslust 111-13

Gawande, Atul 172
generosity 224
Germany, surgical training 182-3, 187
Gladwell, Malcolm 242
gratitude 224-5
gurus 64, 135

hand hygiene 89-94, 98, 147, 239-40, 248
    in the meat packing industry 94-7
handovers xi, 190-1
Hasenboehler, Erik 67-9
Hawthorne effect 92-3
HCAHPS benchmarks 27
hierarchy
    counteracting 241-2
    responsible for poor practice 4-10, 158-9
Hitchcock, Alfred 71
Holmes, Sherlock 41, 79
honesty
    patients 153
    surgeons 42-6, 122-3
hospital-acquired infections 89-90, 103
human error, combating 163-79
Hurlbert, R. John 66

indications for surgery 147-8
infection control (hand hygiene) 89-94, 98, 147, 239-40, 248
informed consent 50, 120
Ingraham, Suzie 132-7

"Janitor Test" 201-2
junior staff 4-10, 83, 146, 149, 158-9
just culture 160

Kissinger, Henry 143
knee, arthroscopic meniscectomy 106-8
Kranz, Gene 240

leadership 177, 237-43
Leriche, René 157
life expectancy 52
limb salvage surgery 82-4, 145-6
listening to the patient 33-40, 128, 150-1
litigation risk 27, 160, 212-16
litter, picking up 238-9
living in the present 217-18

Makary, Marty 115
Malikhin, Anatoly 86
malpractice 125
    examples 110, 118-21
    lawsuits 215-16
Marcus Aurelius 221
maritime collisions 164, 165
Mayo, William 26
McClain, Mike 88, 202, 203
meat packing industry, hygiene in 94-7
media coverage, and the perception of risk 52-3
medical errors xi-xii
    analgesic overdose 12-14
    due to allergies 134, 151
    due to communication failure 35
    leaking aortic anastomosis 4-10
    mortality rates xii, 57, 166-8
    wrong-site/wrong-patient surgery 169-77, 179
meeting a patient before surgery 83, 145-6
melanoma, metastatic 133-7
meniscectomy 106-8

Moore, Ernest E. (Gene) 231-2
Morbidity and Mortality (M&M) conferences 74-7
mortality rates 55, 56, 103
    from medical errors xii, 57, 166-8
music 219

names, using first names 241-2
NASA (National Aeronautics and Space Administration) 161, 174-5, 240
near misses 74, 134
neuroscience of empathy 20
neurosurgery 118-21
Nightingale, Florence 11, 29
no blame culture 160
no harm events 74
nuclear accidents 56

observation bias 92-3
odds (statistics) 48-9
Osler, Sir William 18-19, 33, 217, 224, 231
outcomes 72-3
    improved by empathy 26-7
overwork 83, 85, 207-8, 209-11

painkiller overdose 12-14
Pascal, Blaise 48, 52
paternalism 124, 138
patient advocates 128-37
patient records, electronic 36
patient responsibilities
    engagement with the surgeon 124, 128-9, 138-9, 144-54
    rehabilitation process 139-41, 149
patient safety 166-8
    pre-operative checklists 169-77, 179
    shared decision-making 118-25

perseverance 226
Peters, Thomas J. 181
Pinto, Marc 130-2, 139-42
planning 229-30
Pogo (cartoon character) 248
positive thinking 220-2
postoperative phase 149
    infections 89-90, 103
    rehabilitation 139-41, 149
pre-operative checklists 169-77, 179
probability 48-50
    conditional (Bayesian) 61-4
professional empathy 19
publication bias 67-9
punctuality 197-9

Quality Improvement (QI) schemes 74-8
questioning the surgeon 128, 144-54
    second opinions 129, 131-2, 139, 150

readbacks (teachbacks) 38
reading, bedtime 218-19
Reason, James 174
recreation 231-2
redundancy (fail-safes) 161
rehabilitation 139-41, 149
Relman, Arnold S. 3
respect for others 200
risk
    definition 48-50
    perception of 52-8
    questions about 148-9
rituals 218-20
Robinson, Yohan 187-8

Rockefeller, John 226
role models 81, 237-43
Roosevelt, Theodore 58
Rudolph, Arthur 57

salaries in medicine 85, 114-16
Santiago, José 207-8
Scent of a Woman 29
Schweitzer, Albert 236
second opinions 129, 131-2, 139, 150
seeing a patient before surgery 83, 145-6
self-discipline 218-20
serving humanity 235-7, 250
Sesame Street 21-2
shared decision-making 118-25
shipping collisions 164, 165
Sinclair, Upton Jnr 101
Skolnik, Michael 117, 118-21
sleep deprivation 183-5, 186-9
sleeping patterns 220
Smith, Edward J. 163
Smith, Wade 64, 231
spinal cord injury, steroid use 65-7
spinal surgery 60, 112
spiritual health books 216
standards of care 129
statistics
- being honest with 41-6
- conditional probability 61-4
- risk and odds 48-50

steroid use in spinal cord injury 65-7
stress *see* burnout
sympathy 18
The System culture 84-5, 93-4, 164, 249

systems failures in medicine 166-77
    handovers xi, 190-1

teachbacks (readbacks) 38
terrorism 52-3, 55
test results, keeping track 136
Thompson, Hunter S. 58
time management 219-20, 226-30
timekeeping 197-9
Titanic, RMS 163, 164
titles, not using 241-2
"To Err is Human" (IOM report) 164-6
Tolstoy, Leo 195, 236
training 249-50
    empathy 25, 28, 250
    work-hour restrictions 182-90
triangular osteosynthesis 112-13
Truman, Harry S. 127
truthfulness
    patients 153
    surgeons 42-6, 122-3

uncertainty 59-60, 64
    conditional probability 61-4
    and EBM 65-70
Universal Protocol 169-70
unnecessary surgery 101-4, 147-8
    amputation 145-6
    ankle fixation screw removal 104-6
    appendectomy 108-9
    arthroscopic meniscectomy 106-8
    colloid cyst removal 118-21
    for financial motives 110, 114-16
    Funktionslust 111-13
    for reputational motives 113-14

wait times 197-9
washing hands 89-94, 98, 147, 239-40, 248
    in the meat packing industry 94-7
Weckbach, Sebastian 105
workload
    handovers 190-1
    numbers of operations performed 45, 148, 185-6
    overwork 83, 85, 207-8, 209-11
    surgeons compared with others 85-8
    work-hour restrictions 182-90
wrong-site/wrong-patient surgery 169-77, 179

Zion, Libby 183